THE ECONOMICS OF INSTABILITY

Recovery Beyond Discharge™ and the Cost of Episodic Care

Orlando Andrews

MSLC, CARC, CPRS

Volume Two of the Recovery Beyond Discharge™ Governing Philosophy

First Edition

ISBN: 979-8-9951847-4-4

Dedication:

To the generations who came before,

who carried what was never resolved.

And to the generations who will come after,

for whom solutions are still possible.

TABLE OF CONTENTS

PART III — THE WORKFORCE, INSURANCE, AND EXPOSURE

PART IV — DEMOGRAPHIC COMPRESSION

PART V — INCENTIVE ARCHITECTURE

PART VI — THE DURABILITY STANDARD

PROLOGUE

A Note on Volume One

Many families who love someone struggling with addiction have lived some version of this.

The savings account is drained. Maybe there is a loan against the 401(k), or a family friend comes to the rescue because there is nowhere else left to get the money.

The paperwork is signed. The admissions person sounds certain, and for the first time in longer than anyone can remember, the family lets itself believe: this will be the one that works.

They start talking about next year together as if the person is already in recovery.

They sleep through the night for the first time in months.

Then comes discharge.

The treatment episode is complete. The same person is handed back into the same life that nearly ended them, and the file closes.

Weeks later, the cycle begins again.

Back in the emergency room. The county jail. The same bar stool. Or somewhere no one can find them at all.

And when it happens, the fault lands squarely on the individual.

He didn't follow suggestions.

She didn't want it enough.

They have to reach bottom.

When Systems Let Go made the argument plainly.

If we know people are most vulnerable after treatment, then sending them out with less support and blaming them when they relapse makes no sense.

Relapse is not proof that someone did not want recovery badly enough.

It is often proof that the support ended before the danger did.

And if a system knows this, yet continues to discharge people into the same predictable risk, it is ethically indefensible.

The Economics of Instability establishes the economic case.

Every argument that follows builds from a single structural claim.

Return to use reaches 70 percent within the first year.

Most of that failure happens fast: the majority occurs within the first six months after discharge.

A system in which most people return to use within months of discharge is not producing stability.

It is allowing instability to persist beyond the treatment episode.

When that instability is repeated across millions of lives, it does not remain a clinical problem.

It becomes an economic one.

A system built on cycling people through care rather than resolving instability is economically unsustainable.

The financial consequences of episodic care are not the result of insufficient funding, insufficient compassion, or insufficient clinical expertise.

They are the predictable output of a care framework that treats a chronic condition as though it were acute.

That burden does not disappear when treatment ends. It transfers.

The individual and the family carry part of it.

Hospitals, employers, insurers, courts, and communities carry the rest.

The system has never been required to account for what happens next.

Responsibility ends with discharge, and the accounting stops there.

Volume One asked why the system lets go.

Volume Two asks what letting go costs.

Together, they form a complete argument.

The argument does not begin at the beginning.

It begins where the system ends.

With Jake.

OPENING:

An Ordinary Case

Jake checks his blood sugar before he pours the first drink.

The routine has become automatic. A finger prick. A small drop of blood on the test strip. The number appears on the meter in three seconds.

Tonight, it reads 182.

Higher than he would like. Higher than his endocrinologist would like. Higher than the range associated with the phrase his doctor uses when the numbers improve: "*well managed.*"

Jake sets the meter on the counter beside his insulin pen, looks at it for a moment, and reaches for the bottle of bourbon.

He is forty-eight years old.

From the outside, his life looks stable, or at least functional. He has a job in project management at a regional construction company, a house with a mortgage that is mostly paid off, health insurance through his employer, and a daughter who will begin college applications in the fall.

Jake has three chronic conditions that are technically controlled: Type 2 diabetes, hypertension, and elevated liver enzymes that his gastroenterologist describes as trending in the wrong direction.

His prescriptions are filled for now.

His appointments are kept for now.

His numbers fall within ranges that allow physicians to document the outcome everyone prefers: *"well managed."*

For now.

What the phrase captures is the present.

It does not describe the conditions that produced the present or those the present is reinforcing.

On the kitchen counter beside the meter sits a row of prescription bottles: insulin, a statin for cholesterol, a blood pressure medication, and a small injector pen for Mounjaro, prescribed last year when his A1C climbed to 9.2.

In the cabinet above the stove is a bottle of aspirin his cardiologist added to the list after a stress test produced findings the radiologist described as nonspecific but worth monitoring.

Jake knows the routine.

Most days he follows it.

Not every day.

There are times he slides back into the familiar dissociation.

Some mornings he forgets a dose and makes a judgment call about whether to take it late or skip it. Some weeks he delays refilling a prescription by a few days or even a few weeks. Picking it up requires a trip to the pharmacy, one he keeps meaning to make but hasn't yet.

Some evenings he decides, based on how he feels, that his blood pressure probably isn't as bad as they say and skips the pill before bed.

He is not trying to sabotage himself.

He is living the way people live when they are managing multiple systems simultaneously: the job, the mortgage, the daughter's tuition anxiety, the aging mother in Louisville who calls twice a week with new concerns, and the body that keeps producing numbers that require attention he does not always have the bandwidth to provide.

"Your A1C came back at nine point one. We really need to get that closer to seven, ideally lower. And I notice the ALT is elevated again."

Jake nodded.

He knows what the numbers mean.

Hemoglobin A1C measures average blood sugar across three months. At nine percent, Jake's body has been running far above the range associated with long-term stability.

The ALT elevation indicates stress on the liver. It is not severe, not yet. But the doctor has noted it at each of the last four appointments without seeing the kind of change that would make it stop appearing.

The doctor adjusted the Mounjaro dose.

Jake filled the prescription.

Most of the time he takes it. It's better than the Ozempic, which never seemed to be in stock and was a hassle to fill.

When the doctor asks how the routine is going, Jake answers with a version of the truth.

"Pretty good."

Ten Years Earlier

Ten years before the bourbon and the blood sugar meter and the row of prescriptions on the counter, Jake thought he was simply exhausted.

He was thirty-eight.

He was living, in his own phrase, the full life: late nights, drinks after work several times a week, weekends that rarely ended before midnight.

His circle functioned the same way.

They worked hard.

They drank.

They felt tired.

Nothing about it suggested pathology.

But something about the fatigue felt different.

The thirst was constant, not the ordinary thirst that follows exercise or a salty meal, but an unquenchable, low-grade urgency that no amount of water seemed to resolve.

He urinated constantly.

He woke three and four times a night.

Street signs softened at the edges when he drove after dark.

Words on his computer monitor blurred and sharpened unpredictably.

By the time he told his wife about the symptoms, he had been living with them for six weeks.

She insisted he go to the ER; he chose urgent care.

The nurse ran a finger-stick glucose test, frowned, and ran it again.

The meter returned an error.

A physician stepped in.

"Your blood sugar is too high for our machine to read accurately.

You need to go to the emergency room immediately."

Jake's glucose measured 940 at the hospital.

His body was producing ketones, acids the liver releases when glucose cannot be properly metabolized.

The condition was diabetic ketoacidosis, a life-threatening state that required four days of intensive management before his bloodstream chemistry stabilized.

It was his first hospitalization.

Jake was drinking an average of a liter of bourbon per week at the time, but alcohol was not what brought him to the emergency room.

Diabetes was.

The alcohol was simply present.

It had been present for years.

It was woven into the fabric of the week and normalized by context and repetition until it became invisible in the way things do when they have always been there.

The Attempts to Quit

Jake had tried to stop drinking three times before the diabetes diagnosis and twice since.

In his early thirties, he entered treatment for the first time.

Thirty days. Residential.

Group therapy. A workbook about triggers. A discharge plan and a list of meeting times.

For several months after discharge, sobriety held.

Life felt lighter. His energy returned. His relationships improved.

Then the familiar logic returned.

One drink at a work event.

Then two.

Within three weeks, the old rhythm had reasserted itself.

Over the following decade, Jake repeated some version of that sequence four more times: treatment, a period of sobriety that lasted months rather than years, a gradual drift back toward the bottle, and eventually another attempt.

The treatment episodes themselves were not unusual.

The places appeared on "best treatment center" lists and offered the amenities expected of facilities that worked comfortably with employer insurance plans.

During each thirty-day stay, Jake met once with a psychiatrist for medication management.

At one facility, he worked with a therapist he respected. The conversations felt thoughtful and grounded. After discharge, he would have continued seeing her, but telehealth was not offered. And the program was out of state.

For a few months he kept in touch with several of the men he had gone through treatment with.

The calls and texts were regular at first: updates, encouragement, occasional reminders to go to a meeting and stay connected.

Jake returned to work. Family obligations resumed. The ordinary pressures of maintaining a life reasserted themselves.

Like most things that fade, the contact with his new friends from the program did not end dramatically.

It simply stopped.

Most of the places he attended claimed to have an alumni program

In practice, that usually meant a text message every few weeks.

He is now an alumnus of five different facilities.

At one, there was a staff member trying hard to organize alumni events.

He is no longer there.

The events never happened.

The last facility he chose because they promoted aftercare. He thought that mattered.

When he was discharged, he found out aftercare meant an app.

The app prompted him to rate his mood, cravings, and stress on sliding scales.

If he missed a check-in, it sent a reminder. If he completed it, a dashboard somewhere updated a line on a chart.

It sent motivational quotes regardless of what was happening in his life.

He finds it ironic when “Today is going to be a Great Day” or “One Day at a Time” pops up while he’s drinking.

He answered a call from the last program.
It wasn’t from anyone he recognized.
The voice sounded practiced, almost like a sales call.

The person asked if he was still sober and explained how easy it would be to come back if he needed to.

“There is no shame in admitting you need help.”

He wasn’t sober.
He had no intention of saying so.

He still receives the occasional message from someone at the facilities.

"Checking in. Hope you're doing well."

He replies politely.

"Doing well, thanks."

The exchange is brief, cordial, and functionally meaningless.

Each treatment episode looked like a new beginning. Each produced a period of stability.

None altered the underlying pattern.

The Architecture of Jake's Life

Jake is not dramatic.

He is not collapsing. He is not unhoused. He is not unemployed. He has not lost his family, though the relationship with his daughter is strained in ways neither of them fully acknowledges.

He is not the person who comes to mind when the words alcoholism or addiction are spoken in policy discussions or public health presentations.

He is the person who is not measured in those discussions.

He is statistically common.

Tens of millions of Americans live inside trajectories that appear stable from any single vantage point but reveal slow-motion deterioration across time.

The healthcare framework sees Jake in episodes.

An ER visit.

A prescription refill.

An elevated lab value.

A treatment admission.

A discharge.

Each event is documented, managed, and treated as an appropriate clinical response to a defined presenting condition.

What the model does not capture is the pattern connecting those events.

Only when these episodes are placed in sequence and examined across time does the line become visible: the 940 blood-glucose reading, the 9.1 A1C, the elevated liver enzymes, the blood pressure medication, the stress test result, and the emergency room visit that has not happened yet.

Inside any single appointment, Jake is manageable.

Across time, Jake becomes an escalating problem.

Jake is not a crisis.

He represents a pattern.

He is not the most dramatic case.

He is not the most expensive.

He is the most ordinary.

He represents the tens of millions of Americans managing chronic conditions, cycling through treatment episodes, remaining medically functional by the clinical definition while deteriorating by the practical one.

When trajectories like Jake's unfold across millions of lives simultaneously, the pattern does not remain personal.

It becomes structural.

The American healthcare system is built to respond to crises.

It is not built to manage long-term progression.

And Jake's life, like the lives of millions of others, is just that.

From Medicine to Economics

Long before modern healthcare systems existed, physicians understood something fundamental about illness: many conditions do not resolve through a single intervention.

They unfold across time.

The Hippocratic tradition recognized this reality more than two thousand years ago. The physician's task was not merely to intervene during crisis but to guide the patient throughout the course of an illness. Treatment was not an isolated event. It was a relationship sustained over time, shaped by environment, habit, and the body's capacity to recover.

Chronic conditions were never understood as episodes.

They were understood as processes.

Modern addiction science, neuroscience, and behavioral health research have rediscovered the same principle.

Substance use disorders, like diabetes, hypertension, and cardiovascular disease, unfold across years.

Stabilization during crisis is only the beginning of recovery, not its completion.

Yet the economic architecture of the healthcare system developed in a very different intellectual tradition.

To understand that tradition, it is necessary to turn not to medicine but to philosophy.

In the *Politics* and the *Nicomachean Ethics*, Aristotle drew a distinction that has rarely been applied to healthcare but has never been more relevant.

He distinguished between two modes of economic organization:

Oikonomia and Chrematistics.

Oikonomia, from which the English word economy derives, referred to the management of a household, a community, or a polis in ways designed to sustain the conditions of flourishing across time.

It asked a simple question:

What design allows people to live well over a lifetime?

Chrematistics referred to the accumulation of exchange value through transactions.

It asked a different question:

What is the value of this exchange?

Aristotle did not consider these two modes equivalent.

He regarded chrematistics as subordinate and potentially dangerous when elevated to a governing principle because it optimizes for the transaction rather than for the conditions that allow human life to flourish across time.

A system organized around the maximum number of profitable exchanges can be entirely self-consistent while producing outcomes that are destructive to the population it serves.

The American addiction treatment economy is a chrematistic system operating inside a problem that requires oikonomia.

Addiction is not an acute event.

It is a chronic condition with a biological substrate, a psychological architecture, and an economic trajectory.

Its costs do not resolve at discharge.

They compound.

They spread across institutions.

They move across time.

Whether addiction is interpreted through the brain disease model, the behavioral model, or the social and environmental model is ultimately secondary.

What matters for the design of treatment systems is that it behaves as a long-duration condition whose stabilization unfolds across years rather than weeks.

A system built around short episodes of care will therefore predictably fail regardless of the model used to describe the disorder.

A model that treats admission, the treatment episode, and discharge as a transaction cannot govern a condition that requires continuity, time, and infrastructure to resolve.

The distinction Aristotle drew is not a philosophical preference.

It is the governing economic logic.

Its structural consequence is clear.

A chrematistic treatment model applied to a time-dependent chronic condition will reliably produce escalating cost rather than sustained stability.

The problem is embedded in the model.

When transactions organized around episodes become the governing unit, continuity becomes subordinate, creating a system that cannot reliably produce sustained recovery.

That is the economic frame.

PART I

THE INSTABILITY SYSTEM

Chapter 1:
The Inversion of Prevention

The conventional logic of prevention runs in one direction: toward the child.

If we intervene early enough in schools, in pediatric clinics, and in home visiting programs, we can reduce the behavioral and health consequences that compound over a lifetime.

This logic is not wrong. The research on high-quality early childhood programs shows real returns across educational attainment, criminal justice involvement, and long-term health.

But the conventional prevention frame has a structural blind spot.

It directs attention toward the child while the primary source of the child's risk remains unaddressed.

Children do not generate the instability that shapes their development. They metabolize it. The conditions that elevate a child's lifetime risk originate in the home environment surrounding the child: household addiction, parental mental illness, chronic financial stress, domestic violence, incarceration of a family member.

Adverse Childhood Experiences, the research framework that has reshaped public health thinking over the past three decades, is fundamentally a measure of adult instability transmitted through children.

When a parent cycles repeatedly through treatment and relapse, the child accumulates ACE exposure with each cycle. When a household is destabilized by addiction, every person inside it absorbs that instability: neurologically, emotionally, and economically.

The child who grows up watching a father check his blood sugar and then pour a drink is not simply watching a personal choice. That child is accumulating risk that will shape stress responses, vulnerability to substance use, and the probability of chronic disease across the next forty years of life.

This is the prevention inversion.

Stabilizing adults is the most scalable childhood prevention strategy available. It is not the only strategy. But it is the one the current model most consistently fails to execute. And the failure is not incidental.

The question is not whether instability affects children. It is what continues to produce that instability in the first place.

Because if the source remains unchanged, prevention cannot succeed. The instability it targets is being produced faster than any intervention can contain it.

The architecture of addiction treatment does not interrupt adult instability. It extends it.

In many treatment populations, return to use reaches approximately seventy percent during the vulnerable period following discharge, with substantial recurrence becoming visible within the first six months.

At that rate, the majority of treatment episodes do not produce the durable stabilization required to interrupt ACE transmission to the next generation.

Each relapse cycle increases the probability that a child will accumulate additional adverse childhood experiences.

Each treatment episode that ends at discharge rather than extending through the vulnerable window represents a prevention opportunity that was paid for but not delivered.

The economic consequence of this failure is not abstract. It is measurable.

ACE exposure is widespread across the American population, and its effects extend far beyond childhood. Population-level research links that exposure to substantially higher burdens of depression, chronic disease, heavy drinking, smoking, diabetes, and coronary heart disease.

These are not marginal effects. They represent millions of cases of chronic disease tied to conditions that begin years or decades before the resulting costs become visible.

The financial implications are correspondingly large. Approximately 90 percent of the nearly $5 trillion the United States spends annually on healthcare is associated with chronic and mental health conditions.

A comparative risk-assessment analysis estimated that adverse childhood experiences are associated with approximately $748 billion in annual costs in North America.

For context, a separate peer-reviewed analysis estimated the annual economic burden of child maltreatment in the United States alone at approximately $124 billion.

That $748 billion is already being paid.

It appears across dozens of budget lines in federal, state, and local government. It appears in employer insurance premiums, healthcare system expenditures, disability claims, and criminal justice costs. No single institution sees the full figure. Each sees only its slice. The distributed nature of the cost is precisely what makes it invisible as a unified phenomenon. It is also what makes reform so structurally difficult.

The current system is not designed to make this investment.

It is designed to manage the cost of its own stabilization failure.

A meaningful reduction in ACE exposure would produce a downstream reduction in chronic disease burden on a scale that dwarfs the cost of the adult stabilization programs capable of producing it.

The failure is diffuse. Its costs are spread across schools, child welfare systems, juvenile justice programs, adult treatment centers, and hospital emergency departments. As a result, no single institution bears the full cost, and no single institution has the financial incentive to solve it.

This is not the end of the problem.

It is where the pattern becomes visible.

The child nervously watching from the hallway while his father pours the next drink is not simply witnessing a personal choice.

He is living inside the conditions that allow instability to move across generations.

What produces those conditions and what sustains them is the question that must be answered.

Chapter 2:

The Recurrence Economy

Healthcare costs in the United States have become one of the defining economic facts of modern life.

In 2023, total national health expenditure approached $4.9 trillion. That amounted to roughly $14,500 per person and about 17 percent of gross domestic product.

No peer nation spends anything close to this proportion of its economy on healthcare. Most spend between 9 and 12 percent.

The standard explanation for American healthcare cost exceptionalism focuses on administrative complexity, pharmaceutical pricing, and the fragmentation of care delivery. These factors are real.

But they explain how money moves.

They do not explain why it continues to grow.

The source is chronic disease.

The most expensive conditions in the American healthcare system are chronic. They include cardiovascular disease, diabetes, chronic kidney disease, cancer, chronic obstructive pulmonary disease, Alzheimer's disease, and severe mental health disorders, including substance use disorders.

Together, they account for a disproportionate share of total healthcare spending.

These are not primarily conditions of aging, though age amplifies them. They are conditions that develop slowly across decades, often beginning in early adulthood or even childhood, producing escalating cost as they progress.

To a remarkable degree, their trajectories are shaped by behavioral and environmental factors such as alcohol use, tobacco use, physical inactivity, poor diet, and chronic stress.

What the cost data reveals is that the American healthcare system is not primarily paying for acute care.

It is paying for the long-term management of conditions that developed years or decades before they became clinically expensive.

Emergency departments are expensive. Hospitalizations are expensive. Surgeries are expensive.

But the majority of healthcare spending is not on dramatic interventions.

It is on the slow, continuous management of chronic conditions: the endocrinology visits, the daily insulin supplies, the blood pressure medications refilled month after month, the dialysis sessions three times per week, the home health aides, the memory care units.

Emergency intervention is not the dominant cost in American healthcare. The greater expense comes from managing conditions that persist year after year.

In addiction, that maintenance structure becomes something more specific: a recurrence economy, organized around the same population cycling through the same episodes across years.

The American healthcare system is spending trillions of dollars managing conditions whose origins often lie decades in the past.

From Maintenance to Recurrence

Nowhere is this structure more visible than in addiction treatment.

The addiction treatment industry in the United States is estimated to generate approximately $42 to $45 billion annually.

When mental health services are included, the broader behavioral health sector exceeds $90 billion per year in most industry analyses, though totals vary depending on whether hospital-based psychiatry, outpatient therapy, and ancillary services are included.

The United States currently has 15,953 licensed substance use treatment facilities, as reported in SAMHSA's 2024 National Substance Use and Mental Health Services Survey. Together, these programs form the primary institutional infrastructure through which substance use disorders are addressed.

Although these facilities vary widely in size and specialization, they typically deliver a combination of services that include detoxification programs, hospital-based addiction treatment, residential rehabilitation, partial hospitalization programs, intensive outpatient programs, and standard outpatient counseling.

Taken together, these services form a substantial healthcare sector responsible for millions of treatment encounters each year.

Across the national treatment system, SAMHSA's Treatment Episode Data Set (TEDS) reported approximately 1,498,034 treatment admissions in 2022. Those admissions represent episodes of care rather than unique individuals. A single person may cycle through multiple treatment episodes within a year.

These admissions include detoxification services, inpatient treatment, residential rehabilitation, and outpatient programming across the continuum of care.

From a systems perspective, the addiction treatment economy is therefore not defined primarily by the number of individuals experiencing addiction.

It is defined by the number of treatment episodes delivered each year.

Revenue Per Treatment Episode

When total industry revenue is measured against publicly reported admissions, the economic scale of each treatment episode becomes visible.

The United States addiction treatment market generates approximately $42 billion to $45 billion annually.

Against the 1,498,034 admissions reported through SAMHSA's Treatment Episode Data Set in 2022, that represents roughly $28,000 to $30,000 in industry revenue for every publicly reported admission.

That figure should not be interpreted as a definitive national average price per episode. TEDS does not capture every treatment admission in the United States, particularly admissions occurring in some privately funded programs.

Because private-pay residential programs generally operate at substantially higher price points than publicly funded and lower-intensity outpatient services, inclusion of the full private-pay market would most likely increase the blended average.

The absence of comprehensive national admissions data, however, makes the precise figure impossible to establish.

The comparison nevertheless demonstrates the scale of the economic activity moving through an episode-based system.

Typical treatment costs vary substantially by level of care:

Detoxification programs at $3,000 to $10,000.

Residential rehabilitation at $20,000 to $60,000.

Luxury residential programs at $80,000 to $150,000.

PHP and IOP programs at $5,000 to $15,000.

Standard outpatient counseling at $1,000 to $5,000.

Private-pay residential treatment can substantially exceed the cost of publicly funded and outpatient episodes, with luxury programs reaching well into six figures.

The precise national average is less important than the underlying structure.

Every admission initiates another economic event.

Recurrence Lifetime Treatment Spending

When relapse rates approach 70 percent within the first year after treatment, many individuals experience multiple treatment episodes over time.

A simplified treatment trajectory might look like this: detoxification followed by residential treatment, return to use, then detoxification followed by intensive outpatient treatment, return to use again, then residential treatment, followed by outpatient stabilization.

Each episode represents a new clinical encounter, a new treatment admission, and a new set of healthcare expenditures.

Over the course of several years, total treatment spending for a single individual can easily exceed $100,000 to $300,000.

Importantly, this spending is rarely concentrated in a single intervention.

It is spread across repeated stabilization attempts.

The Structure

At scale, the system reveals its underlying logic.

Revenue is generated through episodes.

Admission initiates the billing event.

Stabilization completes the billable event.

Discharge resets the cycle.

Recurrence regenerates demand.

This is not incidental.

It is structural.

The system is not organized around individuals.

It is organized around episodes.

The Misalignment

Recovery does not unfold in episodes.

It unfolds across time.

Neurobiological stabilization, behavioral change, and environmental restructuring require sustained continuity, not isolated intervention.

The financial structure of treatment is therefore misaligned with the biological reality of recovery.

The system is paid to stabilize.

Recovery requires it to remain.

Instability is not the system's failure condition.

It is the system's output, the predictable result of an architecture organized around episodes rather than outcomes.

Instability returns.

Not as an exception,

but as a continuation.

Because the conditions that produce it remain unchanged.

The system intervenes in the outcome, while leaving the conditions that produced it structurally unchanged.

What follows discharge is not a new problem.

It is the same problem, uninterrupted, continuing along the trajectory the system briefly paused but never altered.

And what continues, reproduces.

Not unpredictably.

Not occasionally.

But with consistency.

The question that follows from this structure is not clinical.

It is economic.

When revenue follows the episode and recurrence regenerates demand in a system organized around transactions rather than trajectories, who is actually bearing the cost of that cycle?

The treatment program is not.

The recurrence produces the next admission.

The insurer absorbs the claims.

The employer absorbs the productivity loss.

The family absorbs the instability.

The federal programs absorb the disability and the long-term care.

The next generation absorbs the ACE exposure.

The cost of the recurrence economy is not paid by the recurrence economy.

It is paid by everyone outside it.

That distribution reveals the economic architecture at work: the cost of episodic failure migrates outward across institutions that never generated it.

The accounting begins here.

Not at the point of treatment,
but at the level of population.

The ACE research does not simply establish individual risk. It establishes population-level disease structure.

Approximately 61 percent of American adults report at least one ACE.

Approximately 16 percent report four or more.

Applied to the current U.S. adult population of roughly 260 million people, this means approximately 159 million adults carry at least one ACE.

Approximately 42 million carry four or more.

These are not small numbers. They are the population under pressure.

The public health modeling that followed the original ACE study attempted to estimate what portion of major disease categories would be prevented if ACE exposure could be eliminated or significantly reduced. The estimates, while imprecise, are directionally consistent.

Approximately 44 percent of depression cases are attributable to ACE exposure.

Approximately 27 percent of COPD cases are attributable to ACE exposure.

Approximately 24 percent of episodes of heavy drinking are attributable to ACE exposure.

Approximately 33 percent of smoking prevalence is attributable to ACE exposure.

Approximately 6 percent of diabetes cases are attributable to ACE exposure.

Approximately 13 percent of coronary heart disease is attributable to ACE exposure.

Sustained adult stabilization could materially reduce ACE exposure across the population.

Consider a scenario in which that exposure were reduced by just 20 percent. A reduction of that scale would prevent millions of chronic disease cases, reduce healthcare utilization across multiple specialties, and produce workforce stability effects that compound across decades.

The implications are not theoretical. The stakes are measured in hundreds of billions of dollars.

Research has estimated that the total economic burden associated with ACE exposure in North America, reflecting costs linked to ACE-attributable health outcomes, exceeds $748 billion annually.

This figure represents costs that are already being paid. They appear across dozens of budget lines in federal, state, and local government.

They appear in employer insurance premiums. They appear in school system budgets and special education expenditures. They appear in disability claims and criminal justice costs.

No single institution sees the full $748 billion.

Each institution sees only its slice: the emergency department sees the acute psychiatric admission, the employer sees the absenteeism, the school sees the learning disability, the criminal justice system sees the arrest.

The distributed nature of the cost is precisely what makes it invisible as a unified phenomenon and what makes reform so structurally difficult.

This distributed invisibility is not a feature of ACE costs alone.

It is the organizing principle of the entire economic argument.

Insurance premium increases, disability claims, nursing home expenditures, and depleted inheritances all exhibit the same distributed invisibility.

Each cost appears on a different institution's balance sheet. Each institution manages its slice. No institution is accountable for the sequence that produced all of them.

That distribution is not accidental.

It is architectural.

And architecture is always a choice.

Four generations are now under simultaneous pressure within that architecture. The window for changing its output is not indefinite.

Chapter 3:

The Demographic Structure

The chronic disease economy does not exist in a demographic vacuum. It is being financed, managed, and absorbed by a population under structural stress, with the burden distributed across generations.

Understanding this structure is essential to understanding why the current moment is different from any previous period in American healthcare history.

The chronic disease burden, the substance use disorder crisis, and the demographic shift toward an aging population are colliding simultaneously within the same generation, producing a compression that no previous healthcare system was designed to absorb.

Baby Boomers — Ages 62 to 80 in 2026

The Boomer generation, approximately 73 million strong, is now between the ages of 62 and 80. The majority have crossed or are approaching the Medicare threshold. They are the largest and most medically expensive cohort in the history of the American healthcare system.

Boomers are entering the peak window for dementia risk. The Alzheimer's Association estimates that more than 6 million Americans currently live with Alzheimer's disease, and that number is projected to approach 13 million by 2050 as the Boomer generation moves through the highest-risk decades.

Long-term care utilization is rising with this cohort. Memory care units are filling. Home health aide demand is increasing faster than the supply of workers trained to provide it.

Boomers are also the generation that will execute the largest wealth transfer in American history to their children and grandchildren over the next two decades.

The condition of that transfer, however, is not simply a function of portfolio performance. It is a function of how much of the accumulated wealth is consumed by long-term care before it can be transferred.

This is not an abstract concern. The median annual cost of a private room in a nursing home in 2024 exceeded $105,000. The average stay before death is approximately two and a half years. For individuals with dementia, the duration of care is typically longer and the cost correspondingly higher.

When chronic disease, including alcohol-related cognitive decline, accelerates entry into long-term care, the asset base available for intergenerational transfer compresses.

The trajectory that begins with a few drinks after work ends, too often, at a nursing home at seventy-two.

Generation X — Ages 46 to 61 in 2026

Generation X, approximately 65 million people, occupies the most structurally complex economic position of any generation in the current moment.

Gen X is the workforce spine of the American tax base. This cohort is in its peak earning years and represents the most productive segment of the employed adult population by experience, seniority, and accumulated human capital.

It is also the generation that is simultaneously financing aging Boomer parents through private caregiving costs and public program contributions, supporting adult Millennial and late Gen Z children through extended financial transitions, and managing its own chronic disease burden.

The alcohol mortality data makes the stakes concrete. CDC mortality analysis consistently shows that the highest absolute concentration of alcohol-attributable deaths in the American population falls among adults ages 45 to 64, placing the heart of the Gen X cohort squarely within that range.

These are not people on the margins of the workforce. They are the people in the middle of their careers, carrying the mortgages, paying the largest share of Social Security and Medicare contributions, and providing the caregiving infrastructure for the generation above them.

When midlife instability concentrates in this cohort, the consequences are not isolated to the individuals experiencing them. They are distributed across the entire economic structure that depends on this cohort's productivity, contributions, and caregiving.

Millennials — Ages 30 to 45 in 2026

Millennials, at approximately 72 million, are the largest adult cohort in the United States. They are the primary generation now parenting young children. Their career trajectories will also shape mid-century economic output.

Absolute alcohol-attributable mortality remains lower among Millennials than among Gen X. This cohort has not yet reached the ages when chronic alcohol exposure produces its largest cumulative mortality effect. Even so, mortality among adults ages 30 to 44 has risen sharply and consistently.

Research published in JAMA Network Open documented steep increases in alcohol-associated mortality among Millennials since 2000, with women in this cohort showing the most dramatic proportional increases.

This pattern matters because it represents the early edge of a mortality curve that will not peak for another fifteen to twenty years. The disease burden accumulating now will appear in the mortality and chronic care statistics of the 2040s and 2050s.

Fatty liver disease, hypertension, and early-stage metabolic disruption are already part of that trajectory.

Millennials are also the generation most affected by the behavioral health conditions that have risen most sharply in the post-financial-crisis, post-pandemic landscape.

Rates of anxiety, depression, and substance use disorder are elevated in this cohort relative to previous generations at the same life stage.

The ACE research implies that some portion of this elevation reflects the childhood experiences of a generation raised during the addiction crisis of the 1980s and 1990s.

Generation Z — Ages 14 to 29 in 2026

Generation Z is just entering the workforce. It is, by most behavioral health metrics, the most stressed generation at entry age in the history of modern polling. Mental health utilization, anxiety diagnoses, and self-reported psychological distress are all elevated relative to previous generations at the same age.

Gen Z represents the future tax base. It will reach midlife in approximately 2045 to 2055. Whether the chronic disease and behavioral health trajectory of this generation diverges from the one set by the generations above it depends, in large part, on whether the adult stabilization infrastructure that would reduce ACE transmission is built in the years immediately ahead.

The window in which that investment has the highest return is now.

The compression is demographic math.

Alcohol-attributable mortality is rising fastest among adults ages 30 to 64, precisely as long-term care demand is rising among those 65 and older.

When mortality accelerates in the economic spine of a population while late-life cost simultaneously rises in the retiring cohort, the fiscal framework faces pressure from both ends simultaneously.

The tax base that finances Medicare is shrinking per retiree. The long-term care cost per retiree is growing. The behavioral health burden in the contributing workforce is rising. And the prevention investment that would reduce the trajectory has not been made at the scale the problem requires.

This is the chronic disease economy under generational pressure.

It is not a crisis in the sense of a sudden shock. It is structural erosion that moves more slowly, remains less visible, and is considerably harder to reverse.

The architecture of the addiction treatment system was built primarily around short episodes of stabilization designed to address acute crises.

But the conditions now driving the chronic disease economy unfold across decades. A system built to respond to episodes cannot stabilize trajectories that develop over time.

Jake is forty-eight years old.

He is not a statistic.

But the problem he embodies is measured in statistics, and those statistics describe four generations simultaneously absorbing the cost of a system that was not built to resolve what it treats.

Chapter 4:
Normalized Risk

There are substances whose dangers are immediately legible. Heroin, methamphetamine, and fentanyl carry risks that are culturally recognized, legislatively codified, and treated as emergency public health concerns when mortality rises.

Policy responses are mobilized. Resources are allocated. The language of crisis is employed.

Alcohol is different.

Alcohol is sold in grocery stores. It is served at corporate events and wedding receptions and holiday parties. It is featured in advertising that associates it with sophistication, relaxation, camaraderie, and success. It is embedded in the rituals of adulthood across virtually every socioeconomic class in the United States.

Its harms are not invisible. Most adults know that excessive drinking is bad for the liver, bad for driving, and bad for behavior. But those harms are normalized in a way that the harms of illicit substances are not.

This normalization is not simply a cultural curiosity. It is an economic and public health fact with measurable consequences.

According to the 2022 National Survey on Drug Use and Health, alcohol use disorder affects approximately 29 million Americans.

That is more than the number affected by all illicit drug use disorders combined.

Yet the treatment gap for alcohol use disorder is among the largest in the behavioral health system.

Only about 7 to 8 percent of people with alcohol use disorder receive any treatment in a given year.

The majority manage their condition, or fail to manage it, without ever entering the treatment system that is supposed to contain the harm.

This is the first way in which normalization distorts the economic picture.

Because alcohol harm is not primarily concentrated in the formally diagnosed and treatment-engaged population, standard metrics undercount it.

The 29 million with diagnosable alcohol use disorder represent the recognized peak of a much larger distribution of alcohol-related risk.

Beneath that peak are tens of millions more who drink at levels that fall below formal diagnostic thresholds but exceed levels associated with health safety. Their cardiovascular risk is elevated, their livers accumulate fatty tissue, their blood pressure is poorly controlled, and their diabetes management is destabilized. Yet they do not appear in addiction treatment statistics because they have not been diagnosed.

Jake is in this population.

He has a documented history of alcohol use disorder, but not at the level his current prescribers recognize or treat as primary.

Instead, he is described in fragments: diabetes, hypertension, elevated liver enzymes.

He has a pattern of alcohol use that interacts with three diagnosed chronic conditions in ways that slowly but measurably worsen all three.

He is not a treatment statistic.

He is a chronic disease cost that has not yet been attributed to its behavioral driver.

The second way normalization distorts the economic picture is through its effect on the class distribution of risk.

Illicit substance use disorders are concentrated, in public discourse and policy, in lower-income and marginalized communities.

This concentration reflects real patterns, but it also reflects surveillance bias. Illicit substance use in wealthy communities is less likely to result in arrest, incarceration, or publicly documented treatment admission.

Nevertheless, the policy response to illicit substance use has historically been organized around communities of concentrated disadvantage.

Alcohol use disorder does not follow this pattern.

Heavy drinking and alcohol use disorder are found across every income level, every educational category, every occupational sector, and every racial and ethnic group.

In some surveys, heavy drinking is more prevalent among higher-income adults than lower-income ones, partly because alcohol is expensive and partly because the social norms of upper-middle-class professional culture normalize drinking in ways that lower-income settings do not always replicate.

This cross-class distribution has two consequences.

The first is political: it makes alcohol a harder target for stigmatizing public health intervention. Policies that effectively demonize illicit drug use encounter far more resistance when applied to substances that are normalized in the constituencies of the legislators voting on them.

The second is economic: alcohol-related instability propagates through the productive core of the workforce. Project managers, accountants, small business owners, healthcare workers, teachers, and executives are all part of that exposure. The economic reach is broader than that of illicit substance disorders that are more concentrated at the margins.

When instability operates in the economic center, the workforce productivity consequences, insurance cost consequences, and tax base consequences are correspondingly larger.

Alcohol is the behavioral risk that spans the entire economic structure.

But alcohol is not the only substance contributing to this instability.

Methamphetamine produces severe neurotoxicity that damages dopamine and serotonin systems, resulting in profound cognitive impairment, psychiatric instability, and long-term neurological decline.

Cardiovascular strain, stroke risk, and systemic organ damage are common consequences of prolonged stimulant exposure.

Opioids produce a different pattern: respiratory depression during overdose events can cause brain hypoxia with lasting neurological damage, and chronic exposure disrupts the brain's reward circuitry in ways that produce long-term anhedonia and emotional dysregulation even after cessation.

Many individuals encounter more than one of these substances across the course of addiction.

The resulting biological damage compounds across systems, affecting the brain, cardiovascular health, endocrine function, immune response, and metabolic regulation.

Neuroinflammation, systemic inflammation, oxidative stress, and mitochondrial dysfunction appear repeatedly across substance categories, each accelerating chronic disease and amplifying long-term healthcare costs.

What distinguishes alcohol within this landscape is not the severity of its damage. Methamphetamine and opioids can produce equally catastrophic outcomes.

What distinguishes alcohol is its reach.

Alcohol is the most widely used psychoactive substance in the United States, the most culturally accepted, and the least likely to trigger intervention until damage is well underway.

It is simultaneously the most widespread behavioral health risk, the least treated substance use disorder, and the most socially normalized.

That combination is not accidental.

It is structural.

And the economic consequences of that structure are proportional to its scale.

Alcohol is not simply another substance within the addiction landscape.

It is the behavioral risk factor most deeply embedded in the economic life of the nation.

The economic case against episodic alcohol treatment extends beyond the fact that alcohol use disorder is undertreated.

When the condition is untreated or inadequately treated, it can accelerate the progression of costly chronic diseases and increase the lifetime cost of managing them.

Consider the interactions.

Alcohol and Diabetes

Alcohol disrupts glucose homeostasis in multiple ways. Heavy drinking can cause both acute hypoglycemia and contribute to sustained hyperglycemia over time. Alcohol impairs the liver's ability to perform gluconeogenesis, the production of glucose during fasting states, creating hypoglycemia risk. It also promotes insulin resistance through inflammatory pathways and contributes to pancreatic damage with chronic exposure.

For someone like Jake who is managing Type 2 diabetes, alcohol use does not simply add a separate health risk. It directly interferes with management of the existing condition.

The glucose variability that alcohol creates undermines the effectiveness of insulin therapy and oral hypoglycemic agents.

It produces readings that are difficult to interpret clinically, contributing to the suboptimal A1C values that Jake's endocrinologist has been managing for years.

The economic consequence is not just more diabetes-related expenditure. It is the accelerated progression of costly diabetic complications such as neuropathy, retinopathy, kidney disease, and cardiovascular disease.

A person managing diabetes without alcohol involvement has a meaningfully different long-term cost trajectory than a person managing diabetes with regular alcohol use, even if neither person's alcohol use is severe enough to trigger a formal treatment episode.

Alcohol and Cardiovascular Disease

Alcohol's relationship with cardiovascular health is dose-dependent in ways that are often misunderstood in popular discourse.

For years, observational research helped popularize the idea that a glass of red wine a day could be good for the heart. That message contributed to the normalization of moderate drinking.

At higher levels, the relationship reverses sharply.

Heavy drinking is associated with significantly elevated risk for hypertension, a leading modifiable cardiovascular risk factor.

It is associated with atrial fibrillation, an irregular heart rhythm that significantly increases stroke risk.

Prolonged exposure can contribute to cardiomyopathy, a weakening of the heart muscle. It elevates triglycerides and disrupts the lipid profile in ways that accelerate atherosclerosis.

Jake's co-occurring alcohol use disorder and hypertension make blood pressure more difficult to manage.

Antihypertensive medications are less effective in the presence of regular heavy drinking.

Compliance with medication regimens is disrupted by the cycle of use and recovery.

The cardiovascular risk trajectory, already elevated by the hypertension, is further accelerated by the alcohol interaction.

Alcohol and Liver Disease

Alcohol-associated liver disease is one of the most rapidly growing causes of liver-related mortality in the United States. It progresses through several stages: alcoholic fatty liver, alcoholic hepatitis, and cirrhosis.

Each stage is more expensive to manage than the previous and more likely to produce costly complications such as liver failure, portal hypertension, and primary liver cancer.

The trajectory of alcoholic liver disease is not primarily determined by the severity of any single episode of drinking. It is determined by the cumulative duration of elevated alcohol exposure over years.

Alcohol use can produce little visible acute harm while sustaining hepatic stress over time. Liver damage can accumulate quietly until it crosses a clinical threshold.

Jake's elevated liver enzymes are the early signal of impending consequences.

The cost is still ahead.

Alcohol and Cancer

Alcohol is a Group 1 carcinogen, classified by the International Agency for Research on Cancer. It is causally associated with cancers of the mouth, throat, esophagus, larynx, colon, rectum, and breast.

The risk increases with dose and duration of exposure. Alcohol is attributable to roughly 1 in every 20 cancer cases in the United States. At current incidence levels, that represents more than 100,000 new cancer cases each year. It also accounts for roughly 1 in every 25 cancer deaths.

Cancer treatment is among the most expensive medical interventions in the healthcare system. The average annual cost of cancer treatment exceeds $150,000 for common cancers, with significant variation depending on type, stage, and therapeutic approach.

Alcohol use disorder can contribute to cancers that might not otherwise have occurred or accelerate cancers that might have appeared years later.

In either case, the economic consequence extends far beyond the treatment cost of the alcohol use disorder itself.

The Multiplier Effect

The significance of these interactions is not simply that alcohol is dangerous in combination with other conditions.

It is that alcohol functions as an economic multiplier.

A person with alcohol use disorder who also has diabetes, hypertension, and elevated liver enzymes does not generate healthcare costs equal to the sum of the four conditions separately.

Each condition is worsened by the alcohol use, and each condition worsens the management challenges of the others. The system is managing a multiplicative effect, not a collection of independent problems.

Episodic treatment may create a period of stability. But when support ends at discharge, the behavioral changes needed to keep co-occurring conditions stable are harder to sustain. The multiplier is not interrupted.

It is paused.

When the alcohol use resumes, the multiplier resumes. And it resumes at a higher baseline of chronic disease burden than existed before the most recent episode began.

Chapter 5:
The Illusion of Containment

Episodic addiction treatment is built on an implicit promise: that the risk brought into a treatment episode will be resolved or meaningfully reduced by the end of that episode.

This promise is not kept, not because treatment providers lack skill or commitment, but because the promise is architecturally incoherent.

Risk does not end at discharge. It continues beyond it.

Addiction alters dopamine signaling, stress response thresholds, and prefrontal inhibitory capacity. Those neurological processes do not normalize within thirty, sixty, or ninety days of abstinence.

Neuroscience research on addiction recovery consistently shows that prefrontal cortex function, impulse control, and emotional regulation continue to improve for twelve to eighteen months after alcohol cessation. Meaningful recovery occurs during that period, but full restoration may extend beyond the timeframes most treatment episodes are designed to address.

A person discharged from thirty days of residential treatment is not a neurologically restored person. They are a person who has been abstinent for thirty days, who has received psychoeducation and therapeutic intervention of genuine value, and whose brain is still in the early stages of a recovery process that will take the better part of a year to produce durable functional change.

At that moment, support withdraws. The structure of the treatment environment falls away at discharge and is replaced by a list of meeting times and an outreach text every few months.

The person re-enters life with a recovering brain and the full weight of the circumstances that preceded treatment.

Within days, the job, the relationship, the financial stress, the family dynamics, the social environment, and the physical environment can all reassert themselves at once.

This is the window in which return to use most often occurs.

The system operates on a timeline that does not match the biology it claims to treat.

The neuroscience establishes the vulnerability window.

What it does not explain is why the system is designed to withdraw precisely at the moment that window opens.

The answer is not clinical. It is not a failure of awareness. The research on neurological recovery timelines has been available for decades. Treatment providers know it. Program directors know it. Insurers know it.

The answer is financial.

When the billing window closes, the support closes with it. Not because the brain is ready. Because the reimbursement cycle is complete.

The end of financial coverage and the withdrawal of clinical support align with the period of maximum neurological vulnerability. That is not coincidence.

The problem is an architectural mismatch.

The economic core of the argument is simple.

The risk profile extends far beyond the period in which intervention is provided.

In the dominant treatment model, intervention lasts for weeks or months.

When intervention duration is shorter than risk duration, risk is not resolved.

It is deferred.

Deferred risk at the individual level becomes an accumulating cost at the population level.

The risk profile for alcohol use disorder does not terminate at discharge.

It continues through the post-discharge vulnerability window, when relapse risk is highest.

The risk continues long after discharge because executive function, impulse control, and emotional regulation may take twelve to eighteen months to meaningfully recover after alcohol cessation.

It continues through the period of identity integration. During that time, a person builds the internal and external architecture of a life that does not require the substance they once depended on.

None of these timelines fits within a thirty-day or even a ninety-day treatment episode.

The treatment field has known this for decades.

The research literature on addiction recovery has documented the temporal misalignment between intervention duration and recovery timeline consistently.

The NIAAA has published guidance indicating that addiction treatment outcomes improve significantly with longer engagement.

The Substance Abuse and Mental Health Services Administration has promoted the concept of that extend support beyond the acute treatment episode.

The National Institute on Drug Abuse has consistently emphasized that addiction is a chronic, relapsing condition requiring ongoing management, and that shorter episodes of care are insufficient for sustained recovery.

Yet the dominant reimbursement structure of the American addiction treatment system continues to organize itself around episodes of thirty to ninety days, with aftercare that is voluntary, sporadically funded, and inadequately resourced to sustain engagement through the high-risk window.

This is not ignorance.

It is incentive alignment.

Episodes are billable in ways that continuity is not. The financial architecture of the system rewards the transaction. It does not reward the trajectory.

Aristotle's distinction returns here with precise force.

A chrematistic system is organized around exchange events, billed episodes, and units of service rendered. It will reliably produce the conditions for the next exchange event.

A recurrence is not a system failure within chrematistic logic. It is the next billable episode.

Oikonomia organizes a system around sustained flourishing across time. That requires different measurement, different reimbursement, and different architecture.

It would require the one-year stabilization investment that the research evidence supports and the current system structurally avoids.

The duration mismatch is not a clinical gap waiting to be closed by new clinical knowledge.

It is the operational expression of a financial architecture that rewards interruption over resolution.

The cost of that interruption can be traced across the institutions that absorb it, the budgets where it appears, and the distance it travels from discharge before becoming visible on someone's balance sheet.

PART II

TRAJECTORY AND COMPOUNDING

Chapter 6:

The Compounding Argument

The Mathematical Fact

Before tracing the economic consequences of episodic addiction treatment across the national balance sheet, a single mathematical fact must be stated clearly enough that its implications cannot be avoided.

In the months following discharge, return-to-use rates across major treatment populations frequently reach approximately seventy percent and higher, with substantial recurrence becoming visible during the early post-discharge period.

The exact percentage varies across studies, substances, and treatment settings. The implication remains the same.

At a seventy-percent recurrence rate, an episode-based treatment system is mathematically structured to expand the instability population faster than it resolves it.

The mechanics of that model are straightforward.

Begin with 100 people who enter treatment for alcohol use disorder.

By the end of six months after discharge, approximately 70 of them have returned to problematic use.

The thirty who have maintained sobriety represent a treatment success rate of thirty percent. For every 100 people treated in a single treatment cycle, the system has yielded thirty stable recoveries and seventy ongoing cases of instability.

Those seventy ongoing cases do not disappear.

They accumulate chronic disease burden during the period of resumed use.

They represent ongoing workforce productivity loss.

They generate insurance claims.

Some re-enter treatment, beginning another billable episode.

If the same recurrence pattern holds, many return to use again within six months, extending the cycle of instability.

Scaling the System

Now scale this across the twenty-one million Americans who need alcohol use disorder treatment in any given year, of whom fewer than eight percent receive any treatment.

The 92 percent who receive no treatment represent an ongoing baseline of untreated instability. That instability contributes to chronic disease, insurance claims, workforce disruption, and public program utilization without ever appearing as an episodic treatment cost because these individuals have never entered the system.

Under the seventy-percent recurrence assumption used here, most of the treated population returns to active use during the six-month modeling window.

The untreated population remains large, while much of the treated population returns to instability before durable recovery is established.

The system resolves only a small fraction of the population it treats in each cycle.

Untreated chronic disease, workforce disruption, adverse childhood experiences, and demographic aging continue to add pressure.

When instability grows faster than the system can resolve it, the gap widens over time.

The system falls further behind with each passing year, not because it is working harder, but because it is working at the wrong problem.

It is managing interruption while the underlying condition continues.

A system with these characteristics is not reducing the instability population.

It is recycling it.

The Hinge

Individual trajectories, repeated across a population, become population-level costs.

What begins as a pattern of individual outcomes becomes an economic one.

At that scale, the problem becomes structural.

The arithmetic, followed to its conclusion, is not complicated.

A nation cannot finance chronic instability through episodic intervention.

Understanding what the numbers show requires no policy position, only a willingness to follow them through and do the math.

The mortality curve that the numbers produce is rising.

But the mortality count is only the most visible expression of a deeper accounting problem.

When a person dies of cardiovascular disease and alcohol use disorder contributed to that death, the death certificate reads cardiovascular disease.

When a person is hospitalized for liver failure driven by decades of alcohol use, the admission is coded as hepatic.

When diabetes complications accelerate by years of alcohol interaction, the claims appear in the metabolic disease category.

Alcohol is the behavioral driver. Present in the disease progression, invisible on the claim.

This is not a documentation error.

It is the structural consequence of a system organized around presenting diagnosis rather than behavioral cause.

Insurance claims do not ask what drove the condition to the threshold that required hospitalization. They record the condition that crossed the threshold.

The result is that alcohol costs are systematically undercounted.

Every institution that absorbs an alcohol-accelerated chronic disease claim believes it is managing a cardiovascular problem, a metabolic problem, a hepatic problem.

No institution is managing an alcohol problem because the alcohol problem has been coded out.

The attribution gap is the distance between where the cost originates and where it appears on the ledger.

That gap is one of the primary reasons the scale of the problem has never produced the policy response its magnitude warrants.

For insurance markets specifically, that attribution gap obscures the full scale of the cost.

Whether the count is seventy thousand, ninety-nine thousand, or one hundred seventy-eight thousand, it represents only the most visible portion of what alcohol-related instability costs the system.

Mortality is the edge of the distribution.

The far larger cost is in the living.

Harm across the population

Consider the structure of alcohol-related harm across the population.

For every person who dies from an alcohol-attributable cause, there are substantially more who are living with the chronic conditions that alcohol has accelerated. The ratio varies by condition: for every alcohol-attributable death from liver cirrhosis, there are many more people with alcohol-related liver disease that has not yet progressed to fatal cirrhosis. For every cardiovascular death with alcohol as a contributing factor, there are far more people managing alcohol-complicated hypertension and cardiomyopathy.

The living population with alcohol-accelerated chronic disease is the dominant cost population.

It is also the population that is most invisible in alcohol policy discussions, because it does not appear in mortality statistics.

The disability cost of alcohol-attributable chronic disease in the United States is estimated at hundreds of billions of dollars annually in direct medical costs, productivity losses, and public program expenditures.

The CDC estimated the total economic cost of excessive alcohol use at approximately $249 billion in 2010, including healthcare costs, lost productivity, crime, and motor vehicle crashes. Adjusted for inflation and the trajectory of costs since then, that figure would be substantially higher in 2026.

The important point is not the precise figure. It is the structure of the cost itself.

The mortality statistics are the visible peak of an iceberg whose mass is almost entirely below the surface, in chronic disease burden, disability claims, workforce productivity loss, insurance premium inflation, late-life care expenditure, and the intergenerational transmission of instability to the next cohort of children who will carry the ACE scores produced by this generation's instability.

Below that visible peak is the slow deterioration of millions of people who are not dying yet but are accumulating the conditions that will eventually require that accounting.

Mortality is the measure the system tracks. It is not the measure of everything the system is already paying for.

The Iceberg

The chronic disease burden flows into the healthcare system as claims. Those claims appear in cardiovascular, metabolic, and hepatic categories rather than behavioral health categories because presenting diagnoses, rather than behavioral drivers, govern how claims are coded.

Those claims drive premium escalation that distributes across every employer and household in the risk pool. The workforce productivity loss flows into employer balance sheets as absenteeism, presenteeism, and turnover.

The disability claims flow into federal programs as SSDI enrollment and early Medicare eligibility.

At each step, the cost travels further from its origin. At each step, the institution absorbing it has less visibility into what produced it.

The iceberg's mass does not stay submerged. Over decades, its costs move through institutional channels that distribute them across the healthcare system, the workforce, the insurance market, the federal balance sheet, and ultimately the household.

That sequence has a structure.

Nonlinear Progression

Chronic disease does not progress linearly. It accelerates.

A person with early-stage alcohol-related liver disease does not accumulate liver damage at a constant rate year over year. The damage accumulates slowly in early stages, then more rapidly as the liver loses functional reserve.

The transition from compensated to decompensated cirrhosis occurs when the liver can no longer maintain adequate function. Once the damage reaches a critical level, that can happen relatively quickly.

The same pattern applies across most chronic conditions that alcohol accelerates. Cardiovascular disease progresses through stages in which early damage is largely subclinical and late-stage disease produces acute and expensive events.

Cognitive decline follows a trajectory in which early impairment is difficult to detect, and late-stage impairment is both severe and expensive to manage.

The economic consequence of this nonlinear progression is that the early years of alcohol-related instability are relatively inexpensive in acute healthcare terms. The medical management costs are modest. The person appears functional and manageable.

But the disease trajectory is being established.

Plaque is building in the arteries. Scar tissue is building in the liver. In the brain, the abnormal proteins associated with Alzheimer's disease are beginning to accumulate. And the insulin-producing cells of the pancreas are being damaged by repeated swings in blood sugar.

These are processes that take place over years and are invisible in the quarterly appointment and the annual labs until they cross a threshold.

When they cross the threshold, the cost accelerates sharply.

A person who has been managing chronic conditions for twenty years at a cost of, say, twelve thousand dollars per year in healthcare utilization does not continue at that rate when the conditions reach a critical threshold.

They may enter a period of intensive management involving hospitalizations, specialty interventions, and complex medication regimens. Annual costs can rise to five to ten times the prior rate.

The episode-based accounting system does not see the twenty-year accumulation. It sees the current year's episode. It manages the current year's crisis. And when the crisis appears medically stabilized, it discharges.

The trajectory continues.

The next threshold arrives.

The next expensive episode occurs.

Incentive Architecture

This is not a problem of inadequate data. The data on chronic disease progression is well-established. It is a problem of incentive architecture.

The financial structure of the healthcare system does not reward sustained investment in continuity that could lower long-term costs. It rewards the management of the crisis when the crisis arrives.

Oikonomia, as Aristotle described it, was concerned with sustaining conditions across time.

Chrematistics was concerned with the value of the transaction at hand.

The American healthcare system, organized around transactions, is generating devastating costs that a system organized around sustainability would have begun managing decades ago.

The consequences eventually reach the household.

Like liver disease, financial damage can accumulate for years before the household appears unstable.

A missed promotion. A higher insurance premium. An occasional treatment episode. Prescription costs for three chronic conditions.

None is catastrophic on its own.

So the household adjusts. It spends more, saves less, postpones purchases, and absorbs losses that rarely appear connected to one another. From the outside, it is still functioning.

But the losses compound. What looks manageable in any single month can become destabilizing across years. Eventually, the household reaches a point of instability.

When the disability claim arrives, or the nursing home placement begins, or the retirement savings prove inadequate, the household does not simply face a larger version of the same problem it has been managing.

It crosses into a qualitatively different financial state that ordinary adjustments cannot reverse.

In medicine, this threshold is called decompensation, the point at which the body can no longer compensate for accumulated damage and the consequences become clinically apparent. Economically, it marks the point at which accumulated instability can no longer remain contained and its costs begin to move outward.

That outward movement has a sequence.

That sequence can be traced step by step and institution by institution, from the acute event through the financial asset that does not arrive.

Chapter 7:
The Capital Flow Sequence

The problem is not simply that the cost moves.

It is that responsibility fragments as it moves.

Hannah Arendt wrote extensively about the conditions under which harm becomes invisible not through conspiracy but through structure, through the fragmentation of responsibility across institutions in ways that ensure no single institution must confront the full scope of what it participates in producing.

In *The Origins of Totalitarianism* and in her analysis of bureaucratic responsibility, Arendt examined how harm can be sustained through distributed participation. Each participant may perform a defined, legitimate function while the system as a whole produces a harmful outcome. Under those conditions, accountability can diffuse to the point of invisibility.

No individual actor is required to see the whole. Each operates within a defined role. The harm persists because no single role is responsible for the full trajectory.

Applied to the economics of addiction and chronic disease, this analysis is precise.

The physician who manages Jake's diabetes does what his role requires. He monitors his A1C, adjusts his medications, refers him to appropriate specialists, and documents the care appropriately.

He does not treat his alcohol use because it is not his specialty, because Jake does not report it as a primary concern, and because the system does not create a financial or structural incentive for him to engage with its long-term trajectory consequences.

The addiction treatment programs Jake has attended also fulfill a defined function. They provided evidence-based clinical intervention, peer support, discharge planning, and alumni outreach.

They won't follow him indefinitely because indefinite follow-up is not reimbursed and because the program's economic model, like all programs in the episodic architecture, is organized around admissions rather than long-term recovery.

The insurance company operates according to its own mandate. It reimburses covered services, manages utilization to control costs, adjusts premiums based on claims experience, and shifts benefit structures when costs rise in ways that expose the company to unacceptable liability.

Jake's employer does what the system requires. They provide health insurance, follow applicable coverage requirements, and do not discriminate against employees because of medical conditions.

Each institution fulfills its role.

The trajectory continues.

This is the mechanism Arendt identifies: harm sustained without malice, without negligence in any individual transaction, through the architecture of fragmented responsibility.

No single institution is required to own the full cost of Jake's trajectory. Each manages only the portion that reaches its ledger. The sequence may begin with an emergency room visit for diabetic ketoacidosis and end years later with a nursing home placement that consumes the assets that remain.

This distributed invisibility is the mechanism through which the capital loop sustains itself.

The economic impact of episodic instability does not stay in one place. It moves through employers, insurance markets, disability systems, government programs, family balance sheets, and ultimately the inheritance a daughter will or will not receive.

The timing differs for every individual, but the pattern of movement is consistent.

The capital flow sequence unfolds as follows.

Acute Event

An ER visit, a hospitalization, an acute medical crisis driven by the interaction of alcohol use and chronic disease. The immediate cost is high and concentrated. It includes emergency department utilization, diagnostic workup, acute management, and sometimes intensive care. These costs are largely absorbed by insurance, with copayments and deductibles flowing to the household.

Work Interruption

The acute event takes the person out of work for a day, a week, or sometimes longer depending on severity. The employer absorbs the lost productivity. The employee absorbs the income loss if paid time off is depleted or unavailable.

Productivity Degradation on Return

The period following an acute event, or following a treatment episode, is typically a period of reduced productivity even for someone who returns to work at full schedule.

Recovery from alcohol-related physiological stress, adjustment to new medication regimens, and the emotional and psychological processing of the event can all reduce functional capacity in ways that may never be formally measured.

Insurance Premium Adjustment

When claims accumulate in an employer risk pool, premiums rise. The premium increase is distributed across all insured employees and the employer.

No single employee sees the full premium consequence of their own claims history, but the aggregate effect of a workforce with elevated chronic disease burden is higher premiums for everyone in the pool.

Insurance Coverage Compression

As premiums rise, employers adjust benefit structures. Deductibles increase. Behavioral health benefits may be restructured through carve-outs. High-deductible health plans become more common. The practical consequence is that treatment, medication adherence, and preventive care become more expensive for the employees who most need them.

Increased Public Program Reliance

As private insurance coverage becomes more restricted, individuals with complex behavioral health and chronic disease needs increasingly rely on public programs.

Medicaid covers an expanding share of behavioral health treatment. Public mental health systems absorb more demand.

Emergency departments can become the default access point for people who cannot obtain care elsewhere, even though they are the most expensive point of care.

Disability Qualification

As the A1C remains elevated, liver enzymes continue trending upward, and cardiovascular risk accumulates, the probability of disability increases.

Disability claims remove people from the workforce, reducing their income contribution, their payroll tax contribution, and their retirement savings accumulation.

They shift financial responsibility from the employer and the individual to the Social Security disability system.

Long-Term Care Entry

The chronic disease trajectory, if not altered, can eventually produce functional decline severe enough to require long-term care. Nursing home care, assisted living, and memory care represent the most expensive phase of the trajectory.

They are financed first through personal assets, then through Medicaid when assets are depleted.

Asset Liquidation

The financing of long-term care through personal assets is not simply an individual financial event. It is an intergenerational economic event.

Assets that would otherwise transfer to the next generation are consumed by care costs. The inheritance is reduced. In many cases it is eliminated.

Generational Capital Compression

The asset liquidation of one generation compresses the starting capital of the next. A daughter who expected to inherit a home, savings, or a financial foundation for her children's education may inherit nothing or only a fraction of what was planned.

Reduced Tax Contribution

Across this sequence, the individual's tax contribution declines. Earlier retirement due to disability, reduced earnings during periods of instability, and lower lifetime earnings from career disruption all reduce the payroll tax, income tax, and Social Security contributions that would have been generated across a full, stable career.

Increased Public Long-Term Care Burden

The combination of depleted assets and extended care needs produces Medicaid-financed long-term care for a growing share of the aging population. The cost shifts from the household to Medicaid, which is jointly financed by state and federal governments.

At each stage of the sequence, financial responsibility shifts. It moves from the individual to the employer, from the employer to the insurance pool, from the insurance pool to public programs, and eventually from the household to the public.

The cost does not disappear. It migrates.

Each institution accounts for the portion that reaches it. None is required to account for the full sequence. None sees the daughter at the end of it.

This is not a series of individual misfortunes.

It is a single economic event, distributed across time and institutions.

The ER visit appears in hospital utilization statistics. The insurance premium increase appears in employer benefit cost data. The disability claim appears in Social Security Administration records. The nursing home placement appears in Medicaid expenditure reports. The reduced inheritance appears in household balance sheet data.

This is precisely the mechanism Arendt describes: harm sustained not through malice or negligence but through a system in which responsibility is fragmented and each participant sees only its part.

An ER physician managing a diabetic ketoacidosis episode does not have visibility into the alcohol use that contributed to the crisis, the treatment episodes that preceded it, the A1C trajectory that preceded those, or the insurance premium consequences that will follow. She manages the episode. The episode is managed correctly. The underlying trajectory is invisible from her position.

The distributed nature of this cost is not merely a measurement problem. It is a reform barrier.

Reform requires the recognition of a pattern. Pattern recognition requires visibility of the sequence, not just the event. An institution that sees only its piece of the sequence has no institutional incentive to invest in solving a problem whose cost it does not fully observe.

This is why recurrence at this magnitude has persisted without generating the level of structural response it would provoke if its full costs were visible within a single sector.

If a single institution bore the full cost of the capital flow sequence, that institution would have an overwhelming financial incentive to invest in the durable recovery infrastructure that would prevent the sequence from completing.

No such institution exists.

The loop continues.

PART III

THE WORKFORCE, INSURANCE, AND EXPOSURE

Chapter 8:

Alcohol and the Employed Adult

The public narrative around alcohol use disorder tends to focus on the visibly disabled, the person who has lost their job, their housing, their family, their physical health.

This narrative, while real, represents only the far end of a distribution that begins long before visible collapse and affects a far larger population.

The majority of people with alcohol use disorder are employed. This fact is both counterintuitive and economically consequential.

The 2022 National Survey on Drug Use and Health found that among adults with alcohol use disorder, approximately 72 percent were employed full- or part-time.

This means that the primary population experiencing alcohol-related health consequences, productivity losses, and treatment cycling is not the marginally housed or unemployed population that dominates the public image of addiction.

It is the working population, the people inside the employer-sponsored insurance model, inside workforce productivity statistics, inside the payroll tax base.

They attend morning meetings. They manage teams. They show up, mostly. They maintain the external performance of stability while the underlying trajectory continues.

Their productivity is lower than it would otherwise be. Their absenteeism is higher. Their healthcare utilization is elevated. Their long-term disability risk is increasing.

None of this is visible in any single quarter's performance review or annual health premium cycle. But it accumulates.

Research on the workforce effects of alcohol use disorder has produced consistent findings across multiple methodologies.

Workers with untreated alcohol use disorders average approximately 14 percent more sick days annually than workers without alcohol use disorders.

They are approximately 2.7 times more likely to experience workplace injury and more likely to file workers' compensation claims.

They generate approximately 50 percent higher healthcare utilization, measured in claims costs, than demographically comparable workers without alcohol use disorders.

When translated into economic terms, the full impairment cost is larger than standard reporting suggests.

The Centers for Disease Control and Prevention estimates that excessive alcohol use cost the United States approximately $249 billion in 2010. It remains the most recent comprehensive national estimate available.

Productivity losses account for approximately 72 percent of that total, reflecting absenteeism, reduced on-the-job performance, and premature mortality among working-age adults.

Standard employer-facing metrics capture only what is directly observable, absenteeism, turnover, and claims.

They do not capture presenteeism, the cost of employees who are present but operating below full capacity, often without detection in standard employer reporting systems.

This is not a semantic distinction. It is the difference between the cost that is measured and the cost that drives the system.

The workforce does not encounter alcohol use disorder as an acute clinical event. It experiences it as diminished capacity over time.

It is also the primary setting in which the early economic effects of alcohol-related instability accumulate diffusely and invisibly, without the triggering events that typically attract institutional attention.

The employees generating these costs are not in crisis. They are at their desks, in meetings, and by every institutional measure that exists, employed and functional.

The system that is supposed to treat them has already discharged many of them and counted them as successes without measuring what happened next.

The concentration of alcohol-attributable harm in the midlife population, specifically the 45-to-64 age range, is not simply a biological curiosity.

It is the economic danger zone.

This cohort represents the highest-productivity, highest-earning segment of the workforce. It carries the largest accumulated human capital of any age group, built through decades of experience, institutional knowledge, and management capacity that cannot be replaced quickly.

It bears the highest tax contribution per worker and finances Medicare through payroll taxes at the same moment it is often supporting aging parents.

When instability concentrates in this cohort through alcohol use disorder, the economic consequences operate at multiple levels simultaneously.

At the individual level, instability produces career trajectory disruption. A period of reduced performance, medical leave, or treatment during the 45-to-55 window can permanently alter lifetime earnings.

At the employer level, midlife attrition, whether through resignation, early retirement, medical leave, or performance-related termination, represents a loss of human capital that is expensive to replace and often impossible to replicate quickly.

At the tax base level, reduced earnings produce proportional reductions in income tax, payroll tax, and Social Security contributions. The compounding effect across the remaining working years of a career is not trivial.

Generation X, the workforce spine of the American tax base in 2026, is the generation that most needs to be stable. It is also the population in which alcohol-attributable mortality is most concentrated and alcohol-related chronic disease most prevalent.

The convergence is not coincidental. It is the demographic expression of a problem that has been expanding for decades.

And its consequences do not remain inside the workforce.

They move immediately into the insurance system, the institution most directly connected to workforce health. It finances the care of the employed population and absorbs the first financial signal of a workforce under pressure.

Chapter 9:

Insurance, Risk, and the Marketplace

When population health deteriorates, the first economic institution to feel it is insurance.

Insurance markets function as risk aggregation mechanisms. Insurers collect premiums from a pool of individuals or employer groups and pay claims as they arise. The pricing of premiums is based on actuarial projections of expected claims. Those projections are calibrated by the health status and risk profile of the insured population.

When the health status of the insured population worsens, claims increase. When claims increase, premiums must rise to maintain solvency. The premium increase is distributed across the pool, not concentrated in the individuals generating the highest claims.

This mechanism means that alcohol-related instability, which produces elevated healthcare claims from the affected individuals, does not remain the financial problem of those individuals alone. It becomes the financial problem of everyone in the risk pool.

The premium signal is therefore one of the earliest and most broadly distributed economic consequences of population-level behavioral health instability.

Long before the disability claims, nursing home placements, and Medicaid expenditures, the cost of instability appears in insurance premiums. Employers and employees absorb those costs without any direct connection to the behavioral health conditions generating the claims.

The scale of employer-sponsored insurance in the United States amplifies this mechanism. Approximately 160 million Americans receive health insurance through employer-sponsored plans.

The employer typically pays the majority of the premium, often 70 to 80 percent for individual coverage and somewhat less for family coverage, with employees paying the remainder through payroll deductions.

Average family premiums for employer-sponsored insurance reached approximately $23,968 per year in 2023, representing an increase of approximately 22 percent over the prior five years. These figures represent a sustained upward trend that has outpaced wage growth consistently over the past two decades.

The premium increase is not driven by a single factor.

But behavioral health conditions, including substance use disorders and their chronic disease health consequences, are among the significant contributors.

Studies of employer insurance claims data have documented that workers with untreated substance use disorders generate healthcare costs that are substantially higher than demographically comparable workers without substance use disorders.

What those studies also document is the specific way in which the accounting for that cost systematically obscures alcohol's role. The claims appear in the premium. But they are not attributed to alcohol. They are attributed to the chronic diseases alcohol accelerated.

That attribution gap is the mechanism that makes the return on investment in durable recovery invisible to the very institutions bearing the cost.

The insurance economics of alcohol use disorder are further complicated by the multiplier.

When an insurance actuary attributes a cardiovascular claim to a person who has alcohol use disorder, the claim is coded as a cardiovascular event. It enters the cardiovascular cost pool. It is analyzed as cardiovascular risk. It produces premium adjustments calibrated to cardiovascular cost trends.

This means that the true contribution of alcohol use disorder to insurance premium inflation is systematically underestimated.

The costs are real. They appear in the premium. But they are attributed to the physical disease categories rather than to the behavioral health condition that amplified those costs.

Effective alcohol use disorder treatment can reduce chronic disease acceleration and the claims that follow. Yet the return on that investment is also invisible in standard insurance accounting.

An insurer who finances a year-long recovery support program rather than a thirty-day residential episode would, at the actuarially expected rate of improved outcomes, see lower long-term claims in cardiovascular, metabolic, and hepatic categories over the following years.

But the attribution of that reduction to the recovery program investment is difficult to establish in standard claims analysis, because the prevented costs are distributed across multiple disease categories and multiple future years.

As insurance costs rise, employers respond with structural adjustments.

The typical employer response to rising healthcare costs follows a predictable sequence.

First, employers increase employee premium contributions, requiring workers to pay a higher share of the total premium.

This is the most straightforward cost-containment measure and the most widely used.

Average employee contributions to family coverage premiums have risen consistently over the past decade, shifting a larger share of the total premium cost onto households.

Second, employers increase deductibles.

High-deductible health plans have become the dominant form of employer-sponsored insurance over the past fifteen years.

Between 2010 and 2023, the share of covered workers enrolled in plans with deductibles above $1,000 increased from approximately 10 percent to more than 50 percent. The typical family deductible for employer-sponsored coverage now exceeds $3,000 per year.

High deductibles do not reduce healthcare costs. They defer them.

Research consistently documents that when people face higher out-of-pocket costs at the point of care, they delay or avoid treatment, including preventive care, chronic disease management, and behavioral health services.

The deferred treatment produces more expensive care later, when the deferred conditions have progressed.

Third, employers restructure behavioral health benefits.

Historically, behavioral health coverage was subject to more stringent limits than medical coverage, including lower session caps, higher cost-sharing, and narrower provider networks.

The Mental Health Parity and Addiction Equity Act of 2008 established stronger parity requirements between behavioral and physical health benefits, with subsequent regulation expanding and clarifying those protections.

But parity in benefit structure does not guarantee parity in access, particularly when high deductibles make all specialty care less accessible regardless of parity requirements.

Evidence suggests that high-deductible plans significantly reduce utilization of outpatient substance use treatment and medication-assisted treatment, both important evidence-based forms of addiction care.

When patients must satisfy behavioral health deductibles before MAT is covered, the financial barrier is greatest at the point treatment could provide the most benefit.

Fourth, and increasingly, employers outsource insurance risk entirely through mechanisms that shift workers from employer-sponsored group plans to individual marketplace coverage.

This development represents a structural transformation in the economics of workforce health, one whose full implications for the working population managing alcohol use disorder are only beginning to be understood.

Individual Coverage Health Reimbursement Arrangements (ICHRAs) represent the most significant structural development in employer-sponsored insurance in the post-ACA period that most workers and most policy analysts have not yet fully absorbed.

Under an ICHRA, an employer provides workers with a fixed dollar contribution, which workers use to purchase individual marketplace insurance plans rather than enrolling in a company group plan.

The employer's healthcare cost becomes fixed and predictable. The worker bears the full variability of individual insurance market pricing, network adequacy, and plan design.

ICHRA adoption accelerated significantly after 2020, when regulatory changes expanded their availability and simplified their administration.

Industry estimates suggest that millions of workers have been shifted from employer group plans to individual coverage, with projections indicating continued growth in adoption among mid-sized employers.

The strategic logic from the employer's perspective is clear: group insurance exposes the company to the collective claims experience of the workforce.

As chronic disease burden and behavioral health claims increase, the resulting pressure is reflected in group premiums across the workforce.

ICHRA structures eliminate that exposure. The employer pays a fixed contribution per worker regardless of what the workforce's actual health experience costs.

The financial consequence for workers is inverse.

Under group insurance, the employer effectively subsidized the health costs of higher-risk workers by spreading those costs across the pool.

Workers with diabetes, cardiovascular disease, or behavioral health conditions paid roughly the same premium as their healthier colleagues because the group pricing mechanism averaged the risk.

Under individual marketplace coverage, the risk pooling is shallower and the plan options more variable.

Workers with complex health needs face more challenging navigation of narrower networks and less predictable benefit structures.

For workers managing alcohol use disorder alongside multiple chronic conditions, the shift to individual marketplace coverage represents a potential reduction in access to the coordinated, continuous care that their health trajectories require.

The employer's financial incentive to invest in workforce health also changes.

Under group insurance, an employer who finances a robust employee assistance program, expands behavioral health benefits, or invests in long-term recovery support for employees with substance use disorders has a financial return on that investment through reduced group claims and lower group premiums.

Under an ICHRA structure, that return disappears.

The employer's healthcare cost is fixed. The workforce health investment that would reduce claims does not reduce the employer's fixed ICHRA contribution. The financial incentive for prevention and long-term stability investment is structurally eliminated.

Chapter 10:
Fiscal Asymmetry

The American federal and state fiscal structure depends on a specific assumption: that a large, stable, productive workforce will generate sufficient payroll tax, income tax, and Social Security contribution revenue to finance the public programs designed to support people who are not in that workforce.

This assumption is under structural stress.

The stress comes from both ends of the demographic spectrum simultaneously.

At the top, an aging Baby Boomer cohort is moving from the role of taxpayer to the role of program beneficiary, consuming Medicare, drawing Social Security, and in increasing numbers requiring Medicaid-financed long-term care.

At the workforce level, the Gen X and Millennial cohorts that are supposed to finance this transition face the behavioral health and chronic disease burden that reduces their productive capacity, their earnings trajectory, their retirement savings accumulation, and ultimately their tax contribution.

The relationship between these two trends is structural. It produces what can be described as fiscal asymmetry, a directional imbalance between two forces moving in opposite directions. Revenue contribution from the working-age population declines while expenditure demand from the aging and disabled population rises.

Payroll Tax Revenue

Payroll taxes, the 6.2 percent employee and employer contributions to Social Security and the 1.45 percent contributions to Medicare, are the primary financing mechanism for these two programs. When the workforce is large and wages are high, payroll tax revenue is robust.

When workforce participation declines, wages stagnate due to chronic disease-related productivity impairment, or workers exit the workforce through disability earlier than their biological age would predict, payroll tax revenue declines.

The alcohol mortality data in the 45-to-64 cohort is directly relevant here. Deaths in this cohort represent not just lost lives but lost years of payroll tax contribution at peak earning levels.

A worker who dies at 54 from an alcohol-attributable cardiovascular event has not contributed to Social Security or Medicare for eleven of the years they would otherwise have contributed. Those are years at the highest earnings level of their career.

The disability pathway represents a parallel mechanism. A worker who qualifies for Social Security Disability Insurance at 51, through the accumulated weight of alcohol-accelerated chronic disease, has transitioned from being a net contributor to the Social Security system to being a net beneficiary.

The fiscal effect is a double negative: reduced inflow and increased outflow.

Income Tax Revenue

Career disruption, earnings trajectory suppression, and early exit from the workforce through disability or early death reduce the lifetime income tax contribution of the affected workers.

The aggregate effect of widespread alcohol-related career disruption across the Gen X cohort is a reduction in income tax revenue during the period when that segment should be generating its highest lifetime tax contribution.

Retirement Contribution

Private retirement savings reduce future reliance on public programs.

A worker who accumulates adequate retirement savings through a full career has lower probability of Medicaid-financed long-term care than a worker whose retirement savings were interrupted by career disruption, medical expenses, or early disability.

The private-to-public cost shift that occurs when retirement savings are inadequate adds to Medicaid expenditure at the back end of the lifecycle.

The three mechanisms operate simultaneously and in the same direction. Each reduces what the workforce contributes. Each increases what the system must absorb. Together they produce a widening fiscal gap that does not correct itself the way cyclical economic pressure does. It widens.

The concrete arithmetic makes the scale visible.

A worker who enters Social Security Disability Insurance at 52, through the accumulated progression of alcohol-accelerated cardiovascular disease and diabetes, generates a fiscal impact that runs in both directions simultaneously.

On the revenue side: that worker will not contribute payroll taxes for the thirteen years between 52 and 65.

At the median earnings level for a Gen X worker in that age range, those thirteen years represent approximately $150,000 to $200,000 in lost payroll tax contribution at peak earning levels.

On the expenditure side: SSDI benefits average approximately $1,500 per month. Over thirteen years that is approximately $234,000 in direct benefit payments.

After twenty-four months of SSDI eligibility, that worker qualifies for Medicare regardless of age, generating Medicare expenditures that the program was not designed to finance for working-age adults.

The combined fiscal impact, contribution loss plus benefit cost plus early Medicare, runs to approximately $400,000 to $600,000 in present value per person.

That is the double negative, stated as simple arithmetic.

Multiplied across the tens of thousands of workers who enter SSDI annually through conditions that alcohol use accelerated, the aggregate fiscal consequence is not marginal.

The Medicare Hospital Insurance trust fund has been projected by Medicare actuaries to face insolvency by the early-to-mid 2030s under current revenue and expenditure trajectories.

This is not a projection of program disappearance. It is a projection of structural imbalance. Incoming payroll tax revenue becomes insufficient to cover projected expenditures without drawing down reserve funds that will no longer exist.

The worker-to-beneficiary ratio tells the story directly.

In 1965, when Medicare was established, there were approximately 4.5 workers for every Medicare beneficiary.

By 2030, that ratio is projected to fall to approximately 2.4 workers per beneficiary, a reduction that reflects both the aging of the Boomer cohort and the behavioral health burden compressing the contributing workforce.

Each worker who exits the labor force through alcohol-accelerated disability before 65 reduces the number of people contributing to the system.

Each beneficiary who enters Medicare earlier through the SSDI pathway increases the number drawing from it.

Over the next decade, that balance will be shaped in part by the treatment architecture decisions being made now.

That is demographic mathematics, not political debate.

PART IV

DEMOGRAPHIC COMPRESSION

Chapter 11:
The Price of Time

The aging of the Baby Boomer generation is the most predictable large-scale economic event in American history.

It was forecast decades before its arrival.

Its cost parameters have been modeled by actuaries, economists, and public health researchers with reasonable precision.

The number of people who will turn 65 each year through 2030 is not a projection. It is a fact about people who have already been born.

What was harder to predict was the health condition in which this generation would enter the years of highest healthcare and long-term care demand. The data is now making that clear.

The Boomer generation did not simply age.

It aged with the health consequences of its behavioral choices across the preceding four decades.

It aged with the accumulated chronic disease burden of decades of tobacco use, alcohol use, and sedentary lifestyles that contributed to the metabolic disease epidemic. Current mortality data now makes the consequences of that alcohol exposure increasingly visible.

It aged with the psychological consequences of high-stress career environments, family disruption, and in many cases untreated behavioral health conditions that were less culturally legible in the 1970s, 1980s, and 1990s than they are today.

The result is a generation entering its most medically expensive decade with a higher chronic disease burden, and in many cases a higher cognitive impairment risk, than the demographic models that designed Medicare and Social Security assumed.

Medicare was designed around expectations about how long beneficiaries would live and how much their care would cost. Both have risen beyond those earlier assumptions.

At the same time, Medicare spending per beneficiary has grown faster than inflation and faster than the payroll tax revenue that helps finance the program.

More beneficiaries are living longer with higher-cost health needs, while fewer workers are contributing to the system. That combination is driving the trust fund depletion projections Medicare actuaries have documented for years.

The gap between what the actuarial models projected and what the Boomers actually cost is a chronic disease burden the models did not anticipate.

A beneficiary who enters Medicare at 65 with well-controlled diabetes and no significant cardiovascular complications generates a meaningfully different cost trajectory than a beneficiary who enters at 65 with poorly controlled diabetes, established cardiovascular disease, early-stage liver fibrosis, and the beginning signs of cognitive decline.

The second profile is not rare. It is the predictable output of decades of inadequately treated alcohol use disorder interacting with chronic conditions across the midlife years.

Cognitive Decline

The most expensive manifestation of that profile, the one that will define the Medicaid and Medicare cost trajectory of the 2030s and 2040s more than any other single factor, is cognitive decline.

Among the chronic disease consequences of alcohol use, cognitive decline occupies a distinctive position in the economics of aging because of the cost structure of its late-stage care.

Dementia, specifically Alzheimer's disease and related dementias, is the most expensive condition in late-life care.

The Alzheimer's Association estimates that the total cost of caring for people with Alzheimer's and other dementias in the United States exceeded $345 billion in 2023 and is projected to rise to nearly $1 trillion by 2050 as the oldest Boomers reach advanced age and Generation X moves through the peak dementia-risk years

These costs are distributed across Medicare, Medicaid, out-of-pocket household expenditure, and unpaid family caregiving.

The Medicaid component is particularly significant because it finances the nursing home care that becomes necessary when dementia progresses to the point where independent living or family caregiving is no longer feasible.

Alcohol's relationship with cognitive health is multidimensional.

Heavy alcohol use over extended periods is an independent risk factor for dementia.

Research published in *The Lancet* and other major journals has linked heavy alcohol use to a significantly higher lifetime risk of dementia. That risk develops through more than one pathway.

Wernicke-Korsakoff syndrome, a severe neurological condition caused by thiamine deficiency associated with chronic heavy alcohol use, represents one of the most direct pathways from alcohol use disorder to cognitive impairment.

With early treatment and nutritional support, the condition can often be prevented or substantially mitigated. Without timely care, it can become profoundly disabling.

A second pathway runs through cardiovascular damage.

Hypertension, atrial fibrillation, and hyperlipidemia are not only cardiovascular risks. They also increase the risk of vascular dementia and contribute to the mixed dementia presentations common among older adults with cardiovascular disease.

The economic implication is straightforward: a person whose cognitive decline is accelerated by decades of alcohol use arrives at the threshold for expensive long-term care earlier than the trajectory without alcohol would have produced.

Each year of earlier long-term care entry represents approximately $100,000 in additional care costs — financed through personal assets first and then through Medicaid when personal assets are depleted.

In a population with widespread alcohol use disorder and high treatment failure rates, the aggregate effect on dementia onset and long-term care timing is not slight.

It is a measurable contribution to the $1 trillion projected dementia care cost of the 2050 demographic moment.

Asset Liquidation

Long-term care is financed in the United States through a distinctive and consequential mechanism: it is primarily paid for through personal asset liquidation, with Medicaid serving as the payer of last resort after assets are exhausted.

Medicare covers limited nursing home stays, typically only short-term post-acute care following a hospitalization. It does not cover the extended nursing home care that dementia and other late-stage chronic diseases require. This care is financed first through out-of-pocket payment by the individual and their family, then through Medicaid when assets fall below the eligibility threshold.

The mechanics of this financing structure create a specific economic dynamic at the household level.

A person who enters nursing home care at 74, rather than at 84, due to alcohol-accelerated cognitive and physical decline will spend up to ten additional years in a care setting that costs approximately $90,000 to $120,000 per year for a private room.

The ten years of additional care represent $900,000 to $1.2 million in care costs that would not have occurred if the trajectory had been different.

These costs are financed through the liquidation of whatever assets the person has accumulated, including retirement savings, home equity, and investment accounts. When the assets are exhausted, Medicaid assumes the cost.

This asset liquidation is not merely a personal financial event. It is a generational economic event.

The home that would have passed to the next generation may instead be consumed by care costs. That equity might have funded a down payment, reduced student debt, or provided the financial cushion that distinguishes households that accumulate wealth from those that do not.

The retirement accounts that would have passed to children or grandchildren are liquidated to finance nursing home fees.

The intergenerational wealth transfer that was expected does not occur. The inheritance that would have shifted the economic trajectory of the next generation arrives diminished or absent.

Across millions of households, this asset liquidation dynamic produces a macroeconomic effect: reduced intergenerational wealth transfer, increased Medicaid expenditure, and the perpetuation of wealth inequality that compounds across generations.

Over the next two decades, an estimated $124 trillion in wealth is expected to transfer from older Americans to heirs and charities, making it the largest intergenerational wealth transfer in American history.

Private wealth management has built sophisticated infrastructure to manage that transfer: trust structures, tax strategy, succession planning, estate litigation frameworks.

What the system has not accounted for is what transfers alongside financial capital.

Trauma can move across generations. Addiction can recur within families. Behavioral health instability can erode the very assets meant to pass forward, consuming home equity, retirement savings, and inherited wealth through the mechanisms described here.

Every family office has a model for inflation risk. Almost none have one for relapse.

The person whose long-term care trajectory was accelerated by decades of untreated or inadequately treated alcohol use disorder did not simply suffer a personal health consequence.

They participated, involuntarily and without understanding the mechanism, in the transfer of family wealth to the long-term care system. Much of that transfer was not inevitable. Durable recovery, sustained early enough and long enough, could have altered the trajectory before instability became disability, long-term care, and finally an exhausted estate.

The cost of failed continuity does not end with the person who needed it. It can consume the capital meant for the generation that follows.

Chapter 12:
Three Generations, One Family

The economic argument is cumulative, revealing distinct mechanisms through which episodic instability translates into fiscal cost across institutions and generations.

Now those mechanisms must be seen together, in the same family, across the same timeline.

The Grandfather

His name is Robert.

He is Jake's father.

He is seventy-seven years old in 2026.

He was exposed to Agent Orange in Vietnam.

At twenty-two, he carried chemicals through jungle heat and did not know they would follow him home.

For decades, the exposure was invisible. His generation called it nothing. We now use terms such as complex PTSD, moral injury, toxic burden, and sustained combat stress to describe what he carried. It settled into his nervous system and his bloodstream.

He came home. He worked. He married. He raised children.

And he drank.

Not theatrically. Not in ways that triggered immediate alarm. He drank the way many men from that war drank, steadily, privately, as if alcohol were insulation against memories that could not be metabolized.

The VA treated him three times over the years.

Inpatient programs in the 1980s and 1990s. Brief stays. Acute stabilization. Discharge when he was no longer in crisis.

Then his wife became ill and convinced him to try again.

After the third admission, he achieved sobriety and held it for five months.

Then she died.

She was the last external structure organizing his days.

The drinking returned.

Explosively.

.His cardiologist tells him clearly:

You have to stop drinking. Your heart will not tolerate it.

He agrees.

There is a pint in the drawer beside his chair, a lot less than the half a liter he was used to.

He does not think of this as relapse.

He experiences it as management.

His medical chart reads like a ledger of cumulative exposure.

Agent Orange–associated risk.
Long-term tobacco use.
Alcohol.
Cardiovascular disease diagnosed in his early sixties.
Multiple coronary stents.
An implantable defibrillator placed when his ejection fraction fell below thirty-five percent.
Hypertension managed by three medications.
Chronic obstructive pulmonary disease.
Early vascular dementia at seventy-one.

When heart failure progressed beyond medication management, a left ventricular assist device (LVAD) was implanted.

Not as a bridge to a heart transplant.

He was not eligible.

Transplant requires documented sobriety.
Sustained stability.
His file could not demonstrate those things.

The LVAD became destination therapy, a machine compensating for a heart weakened by chemistry, stress, age, and accumulation.
He now requires full-time care.

Not institutional placement yet. His daughter has structured her life to prevent that.

She spends $80,000 from her savings and investments annually.

Caregivers rotate through the house.

Social Security covers part.

The VA covers part.

His daughter covers most.

The house he owns remains.

For now.

The Father

Jake grew up in a household shaped less by what happened than by what was missing. His mother would sometimes say that his father had been different before the war. Lighter. More attentive. Capable of humor. Jake does not remember that version of him.

What he remembers is that if his father was not working, he was drinking.

He remembers the sound of him coming in late. The shift in the house before anything was said. The way his mother would move through the kitchen as if nothing had happened.

A few arguments that drew attention from the neighbors.

No interventions.

His mother managed to hide any crisis that would be seen by anyone outside the house.

Her gift was perfection.

And the absence of acknowledgment that any problems existed.

There were no anniversaries marked. No games he can remember his father attending.

No visible affection between his parents. No sense of presence that extended beyond provision.

His mother compensated for it.

She was devoted to the family image. She was at every game, every school event, every performance.

She carried the weight of both roles without naming it. She was, by every external measure, a good mother and later a devoted grandmother.

Why she stayed, he never fully understood.

He learned early what to do with what was in front of him.

Continue.

Don't ask.

Don't name it.

He drinks. Not the way his father drank at his worst, but enough that his physician notes it in the chart, and enough that his wife would make backhanded comments about it.

He provides more than his father did at his age, so he ignores the insults.

His A1C is elevated. His blood pressure is managed with medication.

He has been to treatment before, determined to quit each time.

He stayed sober for a few months, never making it to a year.

Then his mother became ill.

For most of his life, she had been the stabilizing presence, the one who kept things moving, who absorbed what was not acknowledged, who made the house function.

As her illness progressed, that structure began to weaken.

Nothing collapsed all at once.

The progression of his father's hospitalizations, the demands they created, and the tension between him and his sister added to what was already shifting.

So did the stress of his daughter's unemployment and the financial pressure of supporting her.

All of it became more difficult after his mother died.

The drinking returned as it had before, but it was different this time: more persistent, daily.

His wife, now his ex-wife, said something he did not argue with.

"You have a serious drinking problem."

Maya, his daughter, often tells her mom that he's present. But not emotionally available.

The phrasing stayed with him. It was familiar somehow.

He is a project manager at a regional construction firm. He is good at his job.

His performance reviews are satisfactory. His colleagues do not know about the treatment episodes or the continuing pattern.

He knows how to have a good time at Christmas parties.

His employer's insurance covers his prescriptions and medical visits. His diabetes is managed well enough that the endocrinologist does not flag it as an emergency.

To the outside observer, Jake seems stable.

The Daughter

Maya. Jake's daughter. Twenty-three years old now. She graduated from college last year with a degree in communications and a significant debt load from a master's degree she thought she needed.

She is working, living with roommates, trying to establish a career in a labor market that is more complex than the one her father navigated at her age.

She grew up in a household shaped by the trajectories that came before her.

Her parents divorced after years of tension she understood before she had language for it. There were arguments. By the end, they were constant.

They were stressful enough that she learned to read the room. She knew that silence carried as much information as anything that was said.

She lived primarily with her mother, who spoke about her father often, sometimes with frustration, sometimes with exhaustion, rarely without resentment.

She saw him regularly. He came to what was scheduled. He provided what was needed.

But she learned early what it meant for someone to be physically present and emotionally absent.

She was diagnosed with anxiety as a child. It was managed. She watched her grandfather decline.

She absorbed the stress that moved through the household as her father's pattern continued. There were periods when things seemed more stable, followed by times when the instability returned.

She took her first drink at 13. It made her relax.

After her grandmother died, her father seemed different. Even more withdrawn. Quieter but not calmer. Not dramatically. But enough that she noticed.

No one named it.

Life continued.

Alcohol was present. So were prescriptions. Injuries were treated. Pain was managed. Medications were taken, adjusted, refilled.

She learned, without being taught directly, that there were ways to take the edge off what did not settle on its own.

In college, she joined a sorority. The drinking was structured. Social. Expected. Blackouts were not rare. They were discussed casually, compared, laughed about, treated as part of the experience rather than a signal of risk.

She does not identify her relationship with alcohol as a problem. She drinks socially, as most of her group does. She and her physician have both noted the anxiety, but it has not been treated as anything requiring more than a prescription.

Some days she runs.

Some days she drinks.

Some days, when neither running nor drinking is enough, she takes what has been prescribed or something a friend has.

She does not think of it as a pattern.

She thinks of it as what works.

She has never been close to her aunt, who has no children.

They are cordial.

Her aunt is composed.

Precise in a way that does not allow for error.

Everything is handled.

Everything is in place.

But Maya sees the strain.

Her father's sister carries what he cannot.

She does it without collapse, without asking for help, without allowing anything to show.

Maya sees it.

But doesn't have the insight to name it.

Her grandmother had some family money she left to her grandfather.

Her father has not talked about finances.

She knows her grandfather's care is expensive.

She does not know what she will inherit.

Nor does she know that the answer to that question lies in the dysfunction she already carries.

Chapter 13:

Same Family, Different System

The three-generation narrative just described represents one possible trajectory — the one that the episodic treatment architecture most reliably produces.

Now consider an alternative.

In the alternative, Jake's fourth treatment episode, the thirty-day residential program eight years ago following the DUI his employer became aware of, was not followed by alumni check-ins and an occasional text message.

It was followed by a year of structured recovery support, a program that remained in his life long enough to matter.

The difference was not in the quality of the thirty-day episode. The clinical care was similar.

What was different was what happened after the episode ended.

The program did not discharge Jake into silence. It discharged him into a continuing architecture.

A recovery coach called him. Not an app waiting for him to respond, but a person who called.

Every week. For a year.

The calls were structured. They tracked specific things: employment stability, medication continuity, family relationships, stress load, cravings.

When something shifted, the call changed. But the call always came.

Three months after discharge, Jake had a bad week.

He did not call the program.

The program called him.

Not because he had relapsed.

His engagement pattern had changed. He had rescheduled twice. His check-ins were shorter. He had become complacent about working on his recovery goals.

The program was designed to see what he could not see in himself at that moment.

The call did not rescue a person in crisis.

It prevented the return to use pattern that Jake was prone to during disengagement.

There were weekly sessions. Not just focused on substance use, but on the patterns that had shaped it. Family systems. Avoidance. The learned absence he had carried forward without naming.

He was learning more about himself: how he responded to stress, to family dynamics, and to the pressures of his work.

Several months in, he was encouraged to attend a meeting focused on Adult Children of Alcoholics.

He went. Not because he thought it applied to him,
but because he had already worked the steps in AA and didn't feel there was much left for him there.

He felt he had already gotten what he could from the steps.

And this program had twelve more.

He heard his own experience described in language he had never used.

Not the drinking.

The silence.

The not asking.

The not naming.

He was an Adult Child.

It did not resolve everything.

But it changed something.

His medications were managed across the transition. His prescriptions did not lapse in the handoff between the treatment program and his primary care physician because the program coordinated the handoff rather than assuming it would happen.

His diabetes management improved when the alcohol stopped interfering with it.

His endocrinologist noted the change at the six-month appointment.

Over time, his behavior began to change. He noticed when he was leaving conversations without realizing it. He would stop himself. Come back. Ask again.

It was not natural.

It was practiced.

He made it to one year.

Then to five.

Five years into sustained recovery, Jake's chronic disease trajectory changed.

His A1C stabilized at 7.0, a level his endocrinologist was pleased with. His blood pressure normalized on fewer medications. His liver enzymes returned to normal range. The row of prescription bottles on the kitchen counter got shorter.

His career trajectory changed too. Without the productivity drag, the missed days, and the quiet management of the cognitive cost of chronic drinking, the work that had always been there became visible.

He was named Vice President of Operations at fifty — the kind of promotion that had been available to him for years and had kept not arriving.

His earnings roughly doubled. His retirement contributions increased significantly.

His household financial stability, for the first time, was building rather than holding.

His relationship with Maya changed.

Not all at once. Over years.

He began to show up differently.

Not just present. Available.

The difference was not dramatic.

It was consistent.

She noticed.

She did not have language for it.

She did not need to.

She had her father.

The program had built family integration into the architecture.

During one of his father's treatment stays, Jake and Robert participated in family sessions together.

Things that had never been said were said.

Not everything. But enough.

Enough to reduce what had been carried without language for decades.

They continued the work after discharge through telehealth, intense in the early months, processing the grief over his mother's death, then gradually less frequent as the language between them developed.

They discontinued when it was no longer needed. The option remains available.

They haven't needed it.

Robert spent more years at home rather than in care because Jake was stable enough to coordinate his care with his sister.

It was not totally her burden.

She never thought he would be responsible for anything. But here he was.

Jake was able to advocate for Robert with physicians, to really help him see the issues and the effect his drinking was having on his mind and heart.

He said if Jake could do it, he could too.

And somehow Jake was able to get his dad into detox and old-fashioned AA.

He worked the steps and made a veterans' group his home group. He loves it. His sponsor comes by to watch games with him. The LVAD still keeps him inside a lot.

With Dad more stable they were able to manage the financial planning that preserved assets for longer and budget for late-life home health care.

Robert's house was not sold. It was preserved.

When he died at eighty-one, seven years later than the alcohol-accelerated trajectory would have produced, the house passed to Jake.

Jake passed the house to Maya as a foundation, an income-producing asset that could change her financial trajectory.

Maya converted the house into a rental unit.

The income covered what the master's degree had cost her.

For the first time, she was paying down debt rather than accumulating.

A few years into his recovery, Jake suggested she attend an ACA meeting with him. Not because she had a problem.

Because he had begun to understand what growing up in their family had required.

She went. She listened. She heard patterns described that felt familiar in a way she had not named — the tension, the silence, the need to read the room, the way presence and absence could exist at the same time.

She did not experience it as revelation.

She experienced it as recognition.

Around the same time, she began to notice the drinking around her differently.

The repetition. The reliance. The way it moved from occasional to necessary without being named.

She recognized it because she had seen versions of it before. She did not wait for it to become her own pattern.

She had conversations with her father she would not have had before. Not about drinking at first.

About growing up in that house. About what had not been said. About what had been carried without language. He was able to meet her there. Not perfectly. But differently.

She was moved as he included her in his 9th steps for both AA and ACA.

She felt seen.

He was present.

And available.

The difference mattered.

She does not know how close it came to going differently.

She does not know what the years of continued drinking would look like.

She just knows that her relationship with alcohol and her family's reliance on it have resolved.

She knows her father as the person he became.

The divergence between the two timelines is not dramatic in any single moment.

It is architectural.

In the first timeline, we experience the inertia of the status quo.

Each institution, in its moment, does what the existing system asks of it.

The hospital manages the crisis. The treatment program delivers the episode. The insurer manages the claims. The alumni app sends the check-in text. The nursing home provides the care.

Nothing changes.

The trajectory continues.

In the second timeline, the system was designed differently. Not more compassionate.

More structured. A coach who called before the crisis. Medication continuity that didn't assume the handoff would happen.

Family integration built into the program rather than recommended as an afterthought.

Outcome tracking that measured what was accumulating across months, not just what was present at discharge.

One extended investment, a year of recovery support rather than a thirty-day episode, changed the probability of every subsequent event in the sequence.

Not with certainty. But statistically. Across millions of people like Jake, that probability shift produces a different aggregate outcome.

Robert's house.

Maya's foundation.

Her ACE score.

A family system.

None of these are guaranteed by the one-year investment.

But all of them are made more probable by it.

And all of them are made less probable by the architecture that discharged Jake at thirty days and sent a text every few weeks to ask how he was doing.

That different aggregate outcome is the economic argument for durable recovery infrastructure.

It is not an argument about compassion.

The episodic system is staffed by people who are compassionate.

It is an argument about design.

The question is not whether the alternative is possible. A single family across three generations demonstrates that it is.

The question is what standard of design would require it of every treatment organization in the country.

That question cannot be answered at the level of the individual program.

It requires looking at the system as a whole, at how it functions across class, geography, and price point.

Because what emerges, when viewed at that scale, is not variation.

It is consistency.

Chapter 14:
The Classless System

By the time he created the Poor People's Campaign, Martin Luther King Jr. had evolved beyond the argument most Americans associate with him.

It wasn't another Civil Rights March on Washington. It was a poor people's march on Washington.

King was assembling an interracial coalition of economically excluded people, including Black sharecroppers from Mississippi, white Appalachian miners, Latino farmworkers, and Native American communities. He had concluded that the mechanism producing their shared vulnerability was not primarily racial.

It was economic.

By 1967, King was describing a system that protected itself at the top while exposing individuals to risk at the bottom. In practice, it functioned as socialism for the rich and capitalism for the poor.

This was the argument that frightened people more than the dream. Not because it invoked race, but because it didn't.

It named a structural logic that operated across race, across region, across generation. King was no longer asking only why people remained poor. He was asking what kind of economic structure continued to produce poverty in the first place.

Viewed through a systems lens, the implication is difficult to escape.

The system was not failing the poor. It was working exactly as designed.

The addiction treatment system that developed in the decades that followed did not escape this economic divide. It reproduced it.

Luxury residential programs with ocean views, private rooms, chef-prepared meals, and concierge psychiatry.

Premium thirty-day stays that cost more than most families earn in a year. Private coaches and boutique aftercare marketed to the affluent as evidence that their treatment was categorically different.

For those on public programs, the experience looked different. Shared rooms. Institutional meals. Mostly Peer Support. Master's Level Therapists or above often absent. A list of meetings, a discharge plan, and sometimes a follow-up text message.

Though the amenities were not the same.

The architecture was identical.

Admission. Stabilization. Discharge.

Support withdrawn during continued neurological vulnerability.

Success measured at the exit door.

The irony is that what was created to produce better outcomes for one class over time has been shown to produce the same outcome for all.

High rates of post-treatment recurrence are not confined to a single price point, treatment model, or income class. That persistence removes durable recovery from the realm of economic status and places it squarely within structure.

The luxury tier simply packaged the episode differently. There were glamorous magazine layouts, oceanfront campuses, and national television campaigns.

Passages Malibu, one of the most visible luxury programs of the era, became known for an extraordinary promise:

"We don't treat addiction. We cure it."

But beneath the difference in presentation and price, both tiers were selling the same fundamental unit of care.

An episode.

Not durable recovery.

The absence of durable recovery is identical whether the family paid $80,000 or $8,000 for the episode that preceded it.

The industry created a class system of comfort
while maintaining a classless system of failure.

What affluence affords in addiction treatment is not better architecture.

It provides the ability to fill the gaps the system leaves behind. Families with resources can hire a coach or therapist, extend a stay beyond what insurance will cover, or choose an out-of-network program when the in-network option proves inadequate.

Those without the capacity to supplement treatment with some form of structured support are left with respite from an untenable situation and then returned to navigate recovery with limited or no recovery capital.

The underlying vulnerability remains.

What changes is how long a family can absorb it.

For those without resources, the consequences often appear quickly.

Discharge returns them to the same conditions with no financial cushion, no extended support, and little ability to purchase what the system no longer provides.

When instability returns, it is visible almost immediately.

A lost job. An emergency room visit. A return to jail.

And the failure is attributed to the individual rather than to the conditions they were returned to.

For those with resources, the failure is deferred.
Time can be purchased. Extensions can be funded. Consequences can be negotiated. Lawyers get their clients a ticket back to treatment rather than jail.

But the architecture does not change.

The system still withdraws support at the same point.
The trajectory remains the same.

Wealth does not alter the outcome.
It delays when the outcome becomes undeniable.

Robert does not lose his assets all at once.
They are consumed slowly as care costs accumulate year after year.

Jake does not fail to build wealth.

He builds less than he otherwise would have. Year after year, the gap widens until it becomes permanent.

Maya does not inherit what was intended.
She inherits what remains.

And what remains is less.

Not because of a single decision.
Because of a structure that never produced stability long enough for capital to accumulate.

The wealthy family and the poor family are standing at the same threshold.

Wealth did not buy a better outcome. It bought a longer runway to the same outcome.

Generational capital compression operates across every demographic.

The capital flow sequence does not discriminate.

This is the part the system has never been required to account for.

The cost of failing to produce durable recovery does not remain with the person who returned to use. It does not stay within the demographic, the zip code, or the income bracket where it originated.

It moves.

Through emergency departments and insurance premiums.

Through disability claims and Medicaid expenditure.

Through lost productivity and workforce exit.

Through the tax base that absorbs what the system releases.

The employer pays for it in absenteeism and turnover.

The insurer pays for it in premiums distributed across the risk pool.

The federal government pays for it in SSDI enrollment and early Medicare eligibility.

The next generation pays for it in the inheritance that did not arrive.

But no one is outside it.

The executive whose company absorbs the loss.

The middle-class family whose premiums rise to cover claims they did not generate.

The daughter of the wealthy family who discovers that $80,000 bought a temporary reprieve, not long-term recovery.

For someone with few financial resources, being flown to California by a treatment facility that accepted his commercial PPO insurance could feel like winning the lottery.

After discharge, he returned to use and lost his job.

Without the job, he lost the insurance that had made treatment possible and helped support the medical care, therapy, medications, and follow-up that could have continued afterward.

The wealthy family paying privately, the employee relying on commercial insurance, and the person with few resources are all paying for the same architectural failure.

They simply encounter its costs in different forms.

This is where King's final argument becomes most relevant and most urgent.

The Poor People's Campaign was built on a single recognition: the sharecropper, the Appalachian miner, and the Latino farmworker were experiencing different forms of hardship, but those hardships were rooted in the same economic structure.

Race, geography, and circumstance made their experiences look separate, even when the underlying vulnerability was shared.

The movement King was building was not simply asking the wealthy to help the poor.

It was asking people who had been divided by those differences to recognize what they shared, see the architecture beneath it, and act together.

Recovery Beyond Discharge™ is the same argument.

It is not an argument for the poor.

It is not an argument for the marginalized.

It is an argument for every family that has watched the system record success while transferring the responsibility of its outcomes to the individual.
It is an argument to rebuild the architecture made to look like recovery into systems that actually sustain addiction recovery.

And that is where responsibility shifts from the individual to the architecture.

Character, motivation, and individual will are where systems have always been quickest to locate failure. But when the same outcomes repeat across class, price point, program model, and payer, the architecture itself becomes impossible to ignore.

The question is not simply whether the system has failed.

The question is whether it can be redesigned.

And the people with the greatest claim to demand that redesign are not limited to those who lost the most visibly.

They are everyone the system has touched and failed.

Which is most of us.

That is the point.

Programs cycle admissions.

Payers manage episodes.

Institutions remain intact.

The individual does not.

Because the system was not built for continuity.

It was built for throughput.

PART V

INCENTIVE ARCHITECTURE

Chapter 15:
The Chronic Epidemic

The Structural Indictment

A structural indictment has a specific form. It does not argue that the people inside the system are malicious or incompetent. It argues that the system is organized to produce an outcome inconsistent with the purpose it claims.

The structural indictment of the American addiction treatment system is as follows.

Chronic Condition, Episodic Architecture

The system exists to address a chronic condition. It is organized as though the condition were acute.

The distinction between chronic and acute conditions is not merely clinical. It is architectural.

Acute conditions have a defined onset, a defined treatment, and a defined resolution.

A fracture is treated. The bone heals. The treatment episode ends.

The patient's ongoing life does not require the ongoing management of fractures because the underlying vulnerability was resolved by the treatment.

Chronic conditions do not have this structure. They persist across time.

They are managed, not resolved. They require ongoing engagement, not episodes of intervention. Their economic cost accumulates across years and decades, not in discrete events.

Addiction is a chronic condition.

This is not a contested claim.

The American Society of Addiction Medicine, the National Institute on Drug Abuse, the World Health Organization, and the major bodies of addiction research are aligned on this point.

Addiction involves neurological, psychological, and behavioral dimensions that change across time, respond to treatment in ways that require sustained support rather than single interventions, and produce recurrence at rates that are characteristic of chronic conditions rather than acute ones.

Recurrence after treatment is substantial across addiction and other chronic conditions. In alcohol use disorder, major studies document recurrence or failure to sustain abstinence at approximately seventy percent and higher during the first post-treatment year.

Type 2 diabetes after medical management, hypertension after pharmacological control, and asthma after acute intervention, likewise demonstrate why chronic conditions require ongoing management.

No physician treats a patient's hypertension with a thirty-day medication course, discontinues the medication at day thirty on the grounds that the blood pressure has normalized, and then describes the patient as having completed treatment.

The clinical framework for chronic disease management requires sustained engagement, ongoing monitoring, and adaptive response to changes in the patient's condition over time.

The Treatment Contradiction

The contradiction is embedded in the idea of treatment completion.

Addiction is recognized as a chronic condition, but treatment is still organized around episodes with defined endpoints. An individual receives intensive intervention, reaches the end of the treatment episode, and is then described as having completed treatment.

Treatment ends. The condition does not.

The biological and psychological processes underlying addiction continue beyond that endpoint. They still require management, especially in the post-discharge period, when vulnerability is highest.

This is the financial incongruity.

A chronic epidemic managed with episodic architecture is not simply a clinical disconnect.

It is an economic contradiction.
A chronic epidemic managed as though it were acute.

The system produces more recurrence than lasting recovery.

Recurrence generates additional episodes.

The architecture sustains itself in the short term, while producing devastating costs over time.

This is a pattern.

And once a pattern becomes consistent, it becomes predictable.

The word predictable carries significant weight in the ethical and economic analysis of this argument.

It must be defined precisely.

Predictable does not mean certain. It does not mean that every person who completes a thirty-day treatment episode will return to use within six months. Some do not. Their trajectories diverge from the statistical average.

Predictable means that recurrence at a magnitude capable of returning most of a treated population to instability is not an aberration. It is an outcome the system has reason to anticipate.

It is documented across populations and consistent across programs and decades.

Program directors, insurers, policymakers, and other informed actors in the addiction treatment system have had access to this reality for decades.

When an outcome is predictable, continuing to operate the system that produces it is to consent to it.

The word consent here is not accusatory in the conventional sense.

It does not imply that treatment providers intend to produce recurrence.

Most are motivated by genuine concern for the people they serve. They are acting rationally within the systems they operate in.

The consent is structural, not personal.

Incentive Reinforcement

Every billing cycle that rewards an episode rather than a trajectory reinforces the outcome.

Every authorization that approves thirty days but not thirty-one does the same.

Every discharge that occurs because the billing window has closed, regardless of whether stability has been achieved, extends it.

These actions are rational within the financial structures that govern them.

They are rote responses to an incentive architecture that produces predictable outcomes.

But the predictability standard changes the ethical calculation.

Once the aggregate outcome is known, continued operation of the system that produces it is no longer harmless.

It is a decision to accept the outcome, repeated in every billing cycle.

The financial incongruity, a chronic condition managed through episodic architecture, is not a problem of insufficient funding.

It is a design decision. And it requires redesign.

Before redesign can be considered, the cost of the current architecture has to be measured in full.

At scale, recurring instability produces an economic burden that extends far beyond the treatment episode.

The capital flow sequence shows where that burden goes and how it accumulates across the system.

Pattern of Burden

What appears as financial burden is not random.

It follows a pattern.

It appears first in repeated treatment episodes, the cost of cycling individuals through care that does not sustain.

A person who enters treatment three times generates three times the direct cost of one who stabilizes after the first.

It appears as cardiovascular, metabolic, hepatic, and cognitive decline compounds across years of instability, increasing lifetime medical expenditure by hundreds of thousands of dollars per person.

It appears in the workforce, through lost productivity, instability, and disability transitions, producing hundreds of billions in annual economic loss.

It appears in insurance markets, through premium escalation driven by elevated utilization across populations that do not stabilize.

It appears in federal programs as Medicare, Medicaid, and disability expenditures expand in response to chronic disease and long-term care trajectories.

And it appears, finally, in the compression of intergenerational capital, as assets are liquidated, inheritances erode, and economic stability fails to transfer across generations.

No single institution accounts for the full cost.

The system produces it. Consistently.

Across the population affected by alcohol use disorder and related behavioral health conditions, these costs reach into the hundreds of billions of dollars annually.

These costs are already being paid.

They are spread across budget lines that do not identify them as the consequence of episodic treatment architecture.

But they are exactly that.

And eventually, those costs reach the household. They appear in savings that are never accumulated, assets consumed by care, and wealth that never reaches the next generation.

Architecture determines inheritance.

Not as metaphor, but as economic reality.

The design of addiction treatment infrastructure determines what the next generation inherits.
It determines whether stability compounds or erodes, whether

assets are preserved or liquidated, and whether cycles of instability, including adverse childhood experiences, are interrupted or carried forward.

These outcomes are not abstract.

The consequences are measurable across treatment, healthcare, employment, insurance, and public spending.

They are the economic outputs of design decisions made in treatment programs, insurer authorization processes, and policy structures.

When a system is both ethically indefensible and economically unsustainable, redesign is not optional.

It is inevitable.

The question now is how much longer the current architecture can sustain the burden it creates.

Chapter 16:
The Limit of the System

What those costs reveal, when followed to their conclusion, is not scale.

It is limit.

A system that produces this level of distributed economic burden is not merely expensive.

It is operating at the limits of what its design allows.

At that limit, a different conclusion becomes unavoidable: the architecture itself is the constraint.

No amount of effort applied within it will change what it is capable of producing.

The Crisis We Learned Not to See

Before examining the system's structural limits, one question requires an answer.

To date, alcohol kills 178,000 Americans annually, more than double the opioid peak that triggered a $54 billion national settlement and federal legislation.

Why has a condition of this scale generated no equivalent mobilization?

The answer is visible in how two previous epidemics were handled.

HIV/AIDS

The initial response was near silence, not because the mortality was low, but because the affected population was socially marginalized and the harm was concentrated in communities with limited political power.

It took years of sustained advocacy, visible death, and the eventual recognition that the epidemic was spreading beyond its initial population to produce the policy and funding response that ultimately transformed outcomes.

The lesson of HIV/AIDS is that a crisis concentrated among marginalized people can be ignored for years, until the deaths become too numerous, the harm too visible, and the political cost of inaction too great.

The Opioid Crisis

The opioid crisis followed a different path. At its peak, opioid overdose deaths reached approximately 80,000 per year.

The affected population included white, working-class, and middle-class communities whose political representation was higher.

The harm was acute and visible. Overdose deaths are harder to code as cardiovascular events.

The pharmaceutical industry was a traceable corporate actor.

The policy response, when it arrived, was substantial: the SUPPORT Act, expanded MAT funding, state abatement councils, a $54 billion settlement.

Alcohol

Alcohol sits in a different category from both. Its harm is distributed across disease codes. Its affected population spans every demographic and every income level.

The responsible industry spends $2 billion annually on advertising and carries political relationships at every level of government.

And its victims, like Jake, are not dying dramatically.

They are deteriorating slowly, across a decade of elevated A1C readings and trending liver enzymes and managed cardiovascular risk, in ways that are invisible until the crisis arrives.

The policy silence around alcohol mortality is not an accident of oversight.

It is the predictable consequence of a harm that is too distributed, too normalized, and too embedded in the economic interests of a powerful industry to generate the mobilization that its scale warrants.

That silence is part of the architecture.

The reason for that silence is the same reason the economic cost is invisible in any single institution's budget.

The harm appears as liver disease in one chart, as cardiovascular disease in another, as a motor vehicle accident in a police report, as a suicide in a county coroner's record, as an early cognitive decline in a neurologist's note.

No single institution sees the full curve.

Each institution sees only the event that reached its threshold.

This is not coincidence. It is the natural consequence of episodic imagination applied to cumulative harm.

And the architecture cannot sustain itself.

The National Stabilization Equation

The addiction treatment system can be summarized in a simple numerical comparison.

Approximately 46 million Americans meet criteria for substance use disorder. Roughly 20 to 23 million need treatment in any given year.

SAMHSA's Treatment Episode Data Set documents 1,498,034 treatment admissions annually from publicly funded and state-licensed facilities, a figure that does not capture all private-pay programs.

Because national totals including private facilities are not systematically reported, the full volume of treatment admissions across the United States remains only partially measured.

TEDS data indicate that approximately 50 to 60 percent of treatment admissions involve individuals with a prior treatment history, meaning a substantial share of admissions represent repeated episodes of care rather than individuals entering treatment for the first time.

They are the same people cycling back through it.

Long-term recovery infrastructure remains minimal.

Even before considering how many people return to use after treatment, the system is capable of engaging only a fraction of the population requiring stabilization.

But the limited capacity that does exist is not serving only people entering treatment for the first time. Recurrence sends many of those already treated back through the same system for another episode.

Each return draws again on capacity that was already insufficient to meet the need.

The arithmetic becomes unavoidable.

The system cannot reduce instability at scale when recurrence continually feeds demand back into a treatment network already too small to absorb it.

The Economic Transmission Chain

Before examining the system's limits, the path instability takes through the economy should be stated in its compressed form, not institution by institution but as a chain.

Treatment instability
→ chronic disease progression
→ healthcare claims
→ insurance expenditures
→ premium escalation
→ employer cost pressure
→ workforce instability
→ tax base compression
→ federal fiscal exposure

At this point, the cost enters federal programs directly. Medicare, Medicaid, SSDI, and Social Security expenditures rise in response to chronic disease, disability, and long-term care trajectories. These are fiscal costs that accumulate across decades and across millions of individuals.

→ disability enrollment
→ Medicare eligibility
→ long-term care utilization
→ household asset liquidation
→ generational wealth erosion

This is the economic transmission chain, the sequence through which instability moves from an individual health condition into national fiscal consequences.

Each step converts the same underlying instability into a new form of economic loss.

By the time the chain reaches the federal balance sheet, what began as unresolved instability has become a national fiscal liability.

The Disability Pipeline

The pathway unfolds as follows:

Substance use disorder

→ chronic disease development

→ work instability

→ disability qualification

→ enrollment in Social Security Disability Insurance

After twenty-four months of disability eligibility, individuals become eligible for Medicare coverage regardless of age.

Once individuals enter disability status, they rarely return to the workforce.

The fiscal consequences occur simultaneously across three domains: workforce exit, SSDI payments, and Medicare eligibility prior to age sixty-five.

These are not three separate problems.

They are one mechanism producing a fiscal multiplier effect.

The same event reduces the contributor pool, adds to the benefit obligation, and accelerates Medicare enrollment among working-age adults.

Capacity and Recurrence

The structure of the treatment system reflects four fundamental realities: capacity is limited, treatment duration is short, continuity infrastructure is minimal, and recurrence feeds the admission pipeline.

Together these conditions produce a system that functions as a recurrence-driven service economy, in which instability continually regenerates demand for new treatment episodes.

Yet recurrence alone does not fully explain the persistence of instability across the population. To understand that dynamic, it is necessary to examine the capacity of the treatment infrastructure itself.

National Treatment Capacity

Although the United States operates approximately 15,953 licensed substance use treatment facilities according to current SAMHSA data, the majority provide outpatient services rather than residential stabilization.

In SAMHSA's 2024 survey, facility type is reported as services offered, not as mutually exclusive categories, because many facilities provide more than one type of care.

83.8 percent of facilities report offering outpatient care, 22.5 percent residential care, and 7.5 percent hospital inpatient care.

These categories overlap because a single facility may offer multiple levels of care.

Applying these distributions to available capacity data produces an estimated total of approximately 111,083 inpatient and residential beds designated for substance use disorder treatment.

Across a population of roughly 330 million Americans, this translates to approximately 34 designated inpatient and residential addiction treatment beds per 100,000 people.

The limitation becomes clearer when addiction treatment capacity is compared to the broader hospital system.

The United States operates more than 900,000 hospital beds across all medical services.

Yet only about 24,000 of those beds are dedicated specifically to inpatient addiction treatment — roughly two to three percent of total capacity.

This is despite substance use disorder driving emergency department utilization, chronic disease progression, and long-term healthcare spending.

The Capacity Paradox

When this capacity is compared with the size of the addiction population, the structural limitation becomes unmistakable.

At any given moment, less than one-half of one percent of those needing treatment could occupy a residential or inpatient treatment bed.

Even under an idealized scenario in which every residential and inpatient bed turned over once per month, the system's maximum annual residential capacity would be approximately 1.3 million admissions per year, and that ceiling is already close to the total national admissions estimate.

The system has no remaining capacity for the more than 18 million Americans who need treatment and receive none.

Therefore, the current treatment system is structurally incapable of reaching the population experiencing addiction.

Throughput Versus Durability

Throughput describes how efficiently a system moves people through treatment. A person is admitted, stabilized, discharged, and the bed or program slot becomes available for the next person.

Throughput measures movement through the system.

That is different from durability.

Durability asks whether recovery is sustained after the person leaves treatment.

Because capacity is limited, the addiction treatment system has evolved to prioritize throughput rather than durability.

Most resources are concentrated in short stabilization periods.

The resulting cycle is predictable: instability produces a treatment episode, which produces a discharge, the absence of durability (sustained recovery) produces recurrence, which produces another treatment episode.

The system is optimized for the continuous processing of episodes.

It is not optimized for long-term stabilization.

How Capacity Is Actually Distributed

Current treatment infrastructure remains heavily weighted toward short-term stabilization services. The distribution below shows where resources are concentrated:

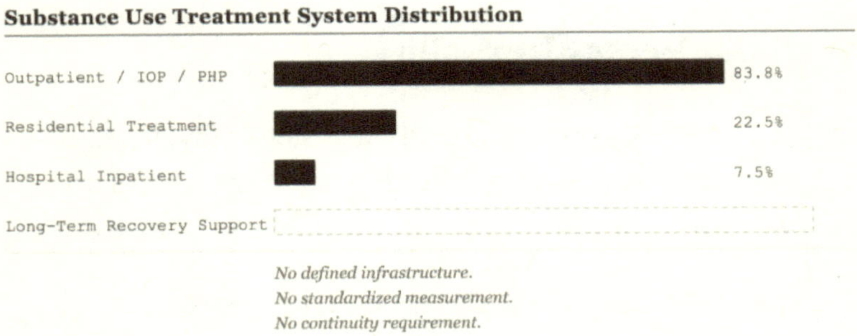

In SAMHSA's 2024 National Substance Use and Mental Health Services Survey, facility type is reported as services offered rather than mutually exclusive categories.

Accordingly, 83.8 percent of substance use treatment facilities report offering outpatient care, 22.5 percent report offering residential treatment, and 7.5 percent report offering hospital inpatient care.

Because a single facility may offer multiple levels of care, these percentages overlap and are not intended to sum to 100 percent.

This distribution reveals the architectural bias of the system.

Most resources are concentrated in acute and subacute stabilization services that bring a person to discharge.

The infrastructure designed to sustain recovery after those phases end remains the smallest and least funded component of the system.

Longitudinal coaching, structured alumni support, and post-discharge engagement remain comparatively limited.

The system maximizes throughput, not durability.

The Insurance Wall

For the fraction of the population that does reach treatment, a second structural barrier awaits, one that has been accelerating quietly, largely outside public discussion.

The shift toward Individual Coverage Health Reimbursement Arrangements has altered the insurance architecture through which workers access care.

The arrangement appears straightforward. Workers have insurance. Employers contribute to healthcare expenses.

But the structure of marketplace coverage differs from traditional employer-sponsored plans in ways that carry significant consequences for the treatment of complex chronic conditions, including substance use disorder.

Most marketplace plans are built around cost control rather than broad network access.

The majority are structured as Exclusive Provider Organizations (EPOs) or narrow-network Health Maintenance Organizations (HMOs).

Unlike Preferred Provider Organization (PPO) plans, these plans typically do not include out-of-network coverage and often restrict care to a defined geographic region.

Many specialized residential programs operate outside the narrow networks used by marketplace insurers, and in some regions, in-network addiction treatment options are limited.

As a result, geography itself can become a barrier to treatment.

A patient may be unable to access a specialized residential program even when it represents the most clinically appropriate level of care, simply because the program falls outside the plan's regional network.

In some cases, a single case agreement may be pursued to authorize out-of-network treatment. But these agreements are rarely accepted, and the approval process is seldom fast enough to meet an immediate treatment need.

Although insurance technically exists, access is extremely limited to the providers available within the plan's narrow network.

Deductibles are often high, particularly for bronze and silver tier plans.

The change in the individual marketplace over the past decade is significant.

In 2014, HMO plans with deductibles of $250 or $500 and PPO plans with deductibles around $1,500 were readily available in the market. Access to major networks was plentiful.

By 2026, newer insurance products increasingly feature smaller networks, PPO options have become far less common, and some marketplace plans carry deductibles approaching $9,000.

Even after deductibles are met, coinsurance structures frequently limit access to residential behavioral health treatment.

Some plans exclude certain levels of behavioral health care from coverage altogether.

Inpatient treatment, residential treatment, and partial hospitalization may be among the services excluded.

When that happens, the cost of that care falls outside the plan's federal out-of-pocket maximum.

Annual out-of-pocket maximums in 2014 were often in the $1,000 to $3,000 range.

By contrast, when needed care is excluded from coverage, there may be no meaningful limit on what the patient can be required to pay.

A policy can therefore advertise an annual out-of-pocket maximum while still leaving a patient with essentially uncapped financial exposure for the treatment they need.

Behavioral health provider networks present an additional challenge.

Even where addiction treatment is technically included within a plan's benefits, behavioral health provider networks are often significantly smaller than networks for general medical care.

Patients frequently encounter long wait times for outpatient behavioral health appointments. Prior authorization requirements can further delay access to care.

The problem is not limited to access. More critically, the financial incentive to improve that access has shifted as well.

The result is not simply narrower coverage.

The architecture shifts more responsibility for access, cost, and continuity onto the individual.

Insurance remains in place, but its protective function has narrowed.

The worker carries more of the risk. The employer carries less.

For a chronic condition that requires sustained access across time, that shift is significant.

It creates another structural barrier to durable recovery.

But the barrier does not end with residential care.

Medication-assisted treatment may still offer another path.

But access to that treatment may require first meeting a deductible approaching $9,000.

The person is insured. The treatment is still financially out of reach.

Structural Inevitability

Taken together, three core dynamics define the system.

The addiction treatment industry delivers millions of treatment episodes annually across a multi-billion-dollar healthcare sector.

A substantial share of those episodes are readmissions, reflecting repeated cycles of treatment.

And the total capacity of the system remains far smaller than the population requiring stabilization.

The central challenge facing addiction treatment is not clinical effectiveness.

It is architecture.

A healthcare system organized primarily around short episodes of care cannot sustainably resolve a condition that unfolds across years or decades.

When recurrence reaches this magnitude, the direction of the system is clear.

It produces more instability than lasting recovery.

That outcome is not the result of negligence. It is the predictable result of an incentive architecture organized around treatment episodes rather than durability.

A system that repeatedly produces recurrence at that scale cannot reasonably be described as a recovery system.

It is a system organized to process episodes while instability continues.

And by this point, the reason is no longer difficult to see.

What Capital Rewards

The consolidation of addiction treatment under private equity ownership has intensified the financial architecture already embedded in the system.

By 2023, private equity owned approximately 7 percent of all licensed substance use disorder treatment facilities nationally, with ownership exceeding 18 percent in several states.

Peer-reviewed research tracking acquisitions from 2019 through 2024, published by RAND, found that privatization of nonprofit treatment facilities was generally followed by increased patient volume and worsening clinical outcomes. The pattern is consistent with a system that rewards more activity without requiring greater durability.

A 2024 analysis in the *Stanford Law Review* concluded that no study to date had found significant improvements in healthcare quality, efficiency, costs, or access resulting from private equity's entrance into healthcare.

Private equity did not create this architecture.

It entered a system already organized around episodes and amplified the variables the system knew how to reward: volume, utilization, occupancy, and financial return.

What remained outside the model was durability.

When financial performance is measured by activity, capital optimizes activity.

When sustained recovery is not measured, it cannot govern investment.

That is the limit.

A system cannot optimize for an outcome it does not require itself to see.

And what it cannot value, it will not build.

Chapter 17:

The Model

.There is a document that describes the American addiction treatment industry with perfect accuracy.

It is approximately forty-seven slides long. It is formatted in a clean sans-serif typeface on a white background with the acquiring firm's logo in the upper right corner.

It was prepared by a team of analysts who worked carefully and well. Every number in it is correct.

Every projection is defensible. Every claim has a source.

It describes a behavioral health platform company operating fourteen residential and outpatient treatment facilities across six states.

It describes the company's revenue per patient day by facility and payer type.

It describes census trends, occupancy optimization opportunities, length-of-stay benchmarks, and EBITDA margins by program level.

It describes the addressable market, including the number of Americans with diagnosable substance use disorders, the percentage currently untreated, and the growth runway that number implies.

It describes the company's competitive positioning, its geographic footprint, its management team's credentials, and its reimbursement mix.

It does not describe what happens to patients after they leave.

Not because the information is systematically tracked and omitted.

Because it is not a variable the model requires.

The document is a behavioral health acquisition deck.

There are hundreds of them in circulation at any given moment, moving between private equity firms, investment banks, and strategic acquirers who together control an increasing share of the American addiction treatment industry.

They are all, in their essential structure, the same document.

They describe a system that is working exactly as designed.

The Analyst

She built the model.

Not this specific model. She has built dozens of them across healthcare services, behavioral health, specialty pharma.

The model is her competency.

She is good at it in the way that people are good at things they have practiced for a decade: automatically, precisely, without having to think about the individual decisions that produce the output.

The model for a behavioral health platform company has a specific architecture.

Revenue is a function of census, length of stay, and payer mix. EBITDA stands for earnings before interest, taxes, depreciation, and amortization. It is used to approximate the operating performance of the business prior to financing and accounting adjustments.
It is derived from revenue after operating expenses, including labor, facilities, and administrative overhead.
Value is then expressed as a multiple of EBITDA.
In behavioral health, that multiple has typically ranged between ten and fourteen times in recent years, reflecting the combination of strong demand and the perceived stability of insurance reimbursement.
At fourteen times EBITDA, a company generating $10 million in EBITDA would be valued at approximately $140 million.
These valuations are not based on demonstrated long-term recovery outcomes.
They are based on the predictability of revenue generated by treatment episodes, regardless of whether those episodes come from new admissions or returning patients.
The model rewards occupancy.
It rewards a payer mix weighted more heavily toward commercial insurance than Medicaid, because commercial plans generally reimburse at higher rates.
It rewards length of stay within the window that insurance authorizes.
It rewards operational efficiency: labor costs per patient day, administrative overhead as a percentage of revenue.

But there is another category the model does not reward at all: sustained recovery.

It does not include a line for six-month post-discharge stabilization rates.

In twelve years of modeling healthcare services transactions, she has never been asked to include one.

The industry knows recurrence exists.
The model has no use for it.
It is built to evaluate the financial performance of a treatment episode business.
Whether the episodes produce durable recovery is a different question.
It is not her question.
Her question is whether the business produces predictable returns.
It does.
The deck is forty-seven slides.
Slide thirty-two shows a sensitivity analysis on EBITDA under different census and length-of-stay scenarios.
Slide thirty-three projects revenue growth over a five-year hold period under base, upside, and downside cases.
There is no slide thirty-four showing what percentage of the patients who generated that revenue are stable one year after discharge.
There is no such slide because there is no such data.
There is no such data because no one built the system to collect it.
No one built the system to collect it because the financial architecture of the industry does not require it.
That is not a gap in the model.
That is the model.

The CFO

He has been the CFO of the platform company for three years.

He manages finance, reporting, and operational analytics across fourteen facilities.

His quarterly board package runs to sixty pages.

It covers census by facility, revenue by payer type, EBITDA by program, labor cost per patient day, and working capital.

It covers key performance indicators: admissions, discharges, average length of stay, bed utilization, and readmissions within thirty days. The last is included because some payers have begun tying modest penalties to thirty-day readmission rates.

It does not cover readmissions beyond thirty days.

It does not cover what percentage of discharged patients are sober at sixty days, ninety days, six months, or one year.

Across its fourteen facilities, it does not track whether former patients are stably employed, securely housed, or engaged in ongoing recovery support.

He knows what the thirty-day readmission rate is because it is on his dashboard. He does not know what the six-month recurrence rate is because it is not.

If you asked him whether the company tracks six-month post-discharge outcomes, he would tell you two things.

First, that the industry lacks standardized longitudinal outcome metrics, which is true.

Second, that the company is actively engaged in value-based contracting pilots that are building toward outcome accountability, which is also true in the sense that one facility in one state is participating in a Medicaid managed care pilot that measures ninety-day engagement rates.

Both statements are accurate.

Neither of them is the same as knowing what happens to patients after they leave.

The board has not asked him for that number.

The board has asked him for census, EBITDA, and payer mix.

Those numbers he has.

Those numbers are good.

The board is satisfied.

The Admissions Director

His name is on a plaque beside the door of the admissions office.

Top Performer, Q3.

He has been in behavioral health admissions for seven years.

He is warm in a way that is genuine, not performed, not trained into him, though the training reinforced it.

He sits with families during the worst conversations of their lives and he is present for those conversations in a way that matters.

He remembers names. He calls back when he says he will.

He has a number.

Fourteen admissions per month.

It is not written into his employment contract in those terms.

It is expressed as a performance expectation, tracked on a dashboard his director reviews weekly, reflected in a compensation structure that includes a variable component tied to admissions volume.

Fourteen.

Some months he makes it easily.

Some months he works the phones on the twenty-eighth and twenty-ninth, reaching back through inquiry lists, following up on families who called two weeks ago and hadn't committed.

Some months he doesn't make it.

The conversation with his director is brief and professional, but he carries it for a day or two before the new month begins.

He recognizes some of the names that come back through.

He has admitted the same person three times in four years.

He doesn't think about it in those terms.

Three times.

Four years.

The same person.

Because each admission is a new encounter, a new intake assessment, a new clinical episode that begins on its own terms.

He is glad each time the person calls.

He tells them it takes courage to ask for help.

He means it.

He does not ask why they came back.

That is not his question.

His question is whether they meet the medical necessity criteria for admission to the level of care the facility provides.

They do.

He completes the admission.

Fourteen.

The Investor Relations Manager

The slide is titled "Outcomes and Quality Metrics."

It shows patient satisfaction scores: 4.7 out of 5, based on surveys administered at discharge.

It shows program completion rates: 78 percent of admitted patients complete the full authorized course of treatment.

It shows a Net Promoter Score of 62, a measure of how likely patients are to recommend the program, which the slide notes is "significantly above healthcare industry benchmark."

It does not show recurrence rates.

It does not show what percentage of the 78 percent who completed treatment are still abstinent at six months.

She presents this slide to limited partners twice a year, at annual meetings and mid-year updates.

The limited partners are pension funds, endowments, and family offices.

They ask good questions.

They ask about the regulatory environment, about the reimbursement landscape, about competitive dynamics in behavioral health.

Occasionally they ask about outcomes.

When they do, she walks them through the slide.

She points to patient experience and program completion as indicators associated with better long-term prognosis.

She positions the company as a leader in the industry's movement toward value-based care.

She assures them that standardized longitudinal outcome metrics do not yet exist at the industry level, so the company focuses on the measures it can track reliably.

The limited partners nod.

They are sophisticated investors.

The metrics before them are familiar: patient satisfaction, completion rates, financial performance.

Long-term recovery is not among them.

They do not ask whether the patients who gave the company a 4.7 satisfaction score and an NPS of 62 are stable one year later.

If they asked, she could not answer.

Not because she is hiding the answer.

Because the answer does not exist in any system the company operates.

What the System Rewards

.Treatment organizations are evaluated using standard financial metrics: revenue growth, margin expansion, occupancy rates, and EBITDA. These metrics reward throughput, payer mix optimization, and operational efficiency.

They do not require demonstration of long-term recovery outcomes. In this framework, a program can improve financial performance without improving durability.

Capital flows toward models that produce predictable returns.

Predictable returns require measurable inputs. When the primary measurable input is the treatment episode, capital will optimize around the episode.

The result is a system in which the most important outcome, whether recovery is sustained across time, is structurally excluded from evaluation.

Including it would require redefining how performance is measured and what revenue is understood to represent.

The revenue itself does not change. What changes is whether $140 million in enterprise value can be treated as evidence of a successful treatment business without asking what happened to the people whose treatment episodes generated it.

So the model stays.

The metric stays.

The long-term recovery outcomes stay invisible.

This is profitable ignorance at the capital level.
It is not the ignorance of people who don't know, but the engineered not-knowing of a system that has arranged itself so that the question never has to be answered.

Those inside the system are not injured by what they don't know.

They are compensated for it.

The analyst does not see the recurrence rate because the model doesn't need it.

The CFO does not see the six-month outcomes because his dashboard was built without them.

The admissions director does not ask why people come back because his job begins at the moment they do.

The IR manager does not have the answer to the outcomes question because the company she represents has not built the system that would produce it.

Each of them is doing the job they were hired to do.

Each of them is compensated for doing it well.

The analyst earns a percentage of the fund's profits when the investment exits. The cleaner the model, the stronger the returns. The stronger the returns, the larger her share of them.

What she is compensated for, precisely, is not asking the question that would force the model to change.

Not knowing, in this architecture, does not cost anything.

It pays.

.

The analyst will raise her next fund.

The CFO will hit his census targets.

The admissions director will make his fourteen.

The IR manager will present the outcomes slide.

The deck will be updated with new occupancy projections and a refreshed market size estimate.

None of them will be in the room where Maya learns that her grandfather's house was sold for his admission to the nursing home and will not be passed down as an asset to her.

The system will record success. The cost will appear somewhere else, as it always does.

And it will keep appearing somewhere else, in the household, in the disability claim, in the Medicaid expenditure, and in the inheritance that does not arrive, for as long as the model is allowed to define what success means.

Because the model does not fail to measure outcomes.

It is not required to produce them.

What it measures, it can claim.

What it does not measure, it does not have to answer for.

And so, the system does not avoid the question.

It removes the need to ask it.

Chapter 18:
Profitable Ignorance

The system does not fail to produce recovery because it lacks knowledge.

It fails because it does not measure what recovery requires.

The architecture of the system is built not only around what it does, but around what it defines as success.

That definition determines what is counted, what is reported, and what is allowed to remain unseen.

Before a system can be held accountable for what it produces, the language through which it defines success must be examined.

Because in this system, measurement does not begin with data.

It begins with words.

Consider four words the addiction treatment system uses routinely.

"Completion."

When a patient finishes a thirty-day episode, the record notes that they have completed treatment.

The word implies a finished process, a state change from incomplete to complete.

But what has been completed? The billing cycle. The authorized episode.

Not the neurological recovery process.

Not the identity reconstruction.

Not the family repair.

Not the accumulation of recovery capital that the research identifies as necessary for durable outcomes.

Using the word completion to describe the end of an episode frames a program as successful before any evidence of recovery exists.

"Aftercare."

The word positions everything that happens after discharge as supplementary, something that comes after the main event.

But the post-discharge period is not after the main event.
It is the main event.

It is the period in which recurrence is most probable, in which neurological vulnerability is highest, and in which the conditions that produced the addiction reassert themselves without a formal structure for recovery.

Calling it “aftercare” is an inversion of rhetoric and clinical reality.

The term carries an implied equation:

care equals recovery.

What follows is therefore something that comes after recovery.

But if use resumes within days or weeks of discharge, what occurred in treatment was not recovery.

Recovery implies stabilization and growth sustained across time.

What occurred was stabilization.

The question is how long it held.

Thirty days?

Ninety?

Until the person walked out the door?

Stabilization is the necessary beginning of recovery.

Stabilization achieved inside a treatment environment is not, by itself, recovery.

And if recovery is still being built, what is called “aftercare” cannot logically be what comes after recovery.

It is the continued care through which recovery develops and becomes durable.

"Relapse"

The word is not unique to addiction. It exists in oncology, where it describes the return of disease after a period of remission.

But there, the meaning is clinical. The relapse belongs to the condition.

In addiction, the meaning shifts.

Because the word implies that a remission occurred and the condition had stabilized before returning.

But if a person leaves a treatment episode and uses within days or weeks, what exactly remitted?

Not the condition.
Not the environment.
Not the underlying drivers across time.

What occurred was not remission.
It was an interruption of use inside a structured environment.

And by naming the return "relapse," the interruption is framed as if it had been a remission, subtly reassigning responsibility to the individual.

The word does not just describe the event.
It protects the architecture from having to account for what it produces.

"Alumni."

The word is borrowed from education, where alumni status follows completion.

A high school student is not called an alumnus after freshman year. A college student is not called an alumnus after completing one year of study. They remain students because the institution's work with them is understood to be incomplete.

Alumni comes later, after the institution's defined course of development has been completed and the person has been instilled with the knowledge, capacity, or competence required to move into the next phase of life or work.

Addiction treatment applies the term differently.

A client can become alumni when a thirty-, sixty-, or ninety-day treatment episode ends, regardless of whether recovery has become durable.

The designation therefore records that the episode ended. It does not establish that the intended outcome held.

That distinction matters because it reveals what the system is actually measuring.

Completion is visible.

Durability is not.

These words are not descriptive.

They are decisions.

They define what the system is allowed to count and what it is allowed to ignore.

Together, they construct a language in which the end of an episode becomes completion, post-discharge vulnerability becomes supplementary care, recurrence becomes individual failure, and the absence of outcomes becomes evidence of success.

This is not simply a failure of measurement.

It is a distortion of the standard itself.

A system that has designed its way out of measuring what it produces can define success at discharge and remain unaccountable for what happens after it.

The Limits of Measurement

The problem, then, is not simply that the system fails to measure recovery across time.

It is that the system makes claims about recovery using evidence gathered almost entirely within the treatment episode.

The question is what those measurements entitle the system to claim.

Kant provides the framework for answering that question.

In the *Critique of Pure Reason*, Immanuel Kant established a boundary that has been applied to epistemology but rarely to institutional economics.

In its classical form, Kant's argument concerns the limits of human knowledge.

In modern institutional systems, that same question can be applied to the boundaries created by measurement.

A system cannot claim to know what it has not measured.

More precisely: a system cannot claim authority over conclusions it has reached while excluding the evidence necessary to test them.

And when that limit is designed rather than accidental, the problem is no longer merely intellectual.

It becomes a moral one.

A system that asserts conclusions while selectively ignoring the evidence that would complicate those conclusions has forfeited the legitimacy of its claims.

Applied to addiction treatment, the Kantian critique is precise and devastating.

Addiction treatment systems claim to produce recovery.

Recovery, by any reasonable definition, is a condition that persists beyond the point of discharge, a stabilization of health, behavior, relationships, and economic function across time.

Recovery is not defined within the walls of a treatment program.

It is defined in the life that follows.

But recovery systems, as currently designed, do not measure what happens in the life that follows.

They measure what happens inside the treatment episode.

They measure admissions. They measure length of stay. They measure program completion. They measure abstinence at discharge.

They measure readmissions but only the readmissions that return to their own program and only within the timeframes that payers define as relevant.

They do not measure what happens to the person who completes the program and does not return.

They do not measure the trajectory of recovery capital in the months and years after discharge.

They do not measure chronic disease progression in former clients.

They do not measure workforce stability, family stability, or economic stability in the two or five or ten years following treatment.

Everything the system measures is concentrated around the episode itself: entry, participation, completion, discharge.

What happens after the person leaves falls outside the frame.

In essence, they measure the doorway.

They do not measure the building.

The Inconvenient Truth

The period outside the treatment episode is not a statistical afterthought.

It is where much of the outcome becomes visible.

Opioids

For opioid use disorder, the post-treatment vulnerability can be immediate and severe.

Following inpatient opioid detoxification, one prospective study found that 91 percent of participants relapsed after discharge, with 59 percent experiencing their initial relapse within the first week.

Other research examining opioid detox and residential treatment has documented recurrence above seventy percent and, in some populations, into the eighty- and ninety-percent range during the months following treatment.

Methamphetamine

Methamphetamine produces the same structural problem through a different pattern.

The recurrence data reflect that instability.

In one longitudinal study of 350 people treated for methamphetamine dependence, 61 percent returned to use within the first year after discharge.

In a separate residential rehabilitation cohort, 77 percent did not maintain continuous abstinence through one year.

Different samples, different measures, but the same structural pattern: instability remains high well beyond the treatment episode.

Across follow-up periods extending to approximately five years, recurrence continues to accumulate, showing that instability can persist long after the treatment episode has ended.

Alcohol

Then there is alcohol.

Alcohol matters differently because it is not confined to a visibly marginalized population.

It is embedded in the workforce.

In families.

In employer-sponsored insurance.

In professional life.

In the chronic disease economy.

And in the economic model itself.

The treatment evidence is correspondingly important.

In Project MATCH, one of the largest alcohol treatment studies ever conducted, approximately 75 percent of participants resumed drinking during the twelve months following treatment.

A separate analysis of the Project MATCH outpatient population found that roughly three-quarters experienced at least some heavy drinking during the first post-treatment year.

The COMBINE study, an NIAAA-sponsored randomized trial involving 1,383 alcohol-dependent adults across eleven academic sites in the United States, produced an equally consequential result.

During the twelve months after active treatment ended, between approximately 77.5 and 86.6 percent of participants across the individual treatment groups experienced at least one heavy-drinking day.

The interventions differed.

The medications differed.

The behavioral treatment differed.

The intensity of medical management differed.

Yet by one year after treatment, the differences between treatment groups were no longer statistically significant.

Across the trial, the overwhelming majority had experienced heavy drinking again.

Different studies define recurrence differently.

Some measure any return to use.

Some measure heavy use.

Some measure continuous abstinence.

Some examine people following detoxification.

Others examine residential or outpatient treatment.

Those distinctions matter.

These findings are not interchangeable statistics, and they should not be treated as though they are.

But they establish the same structural fact.

The magnitude of post-treatment instability is not a marginal finding.

Across major substance-use populations, recurrence or failure to sustain abstinence repeatedly reaches seventy percent and higher.

Sometimes substantially higher.

A seventy-percent recurrence assumption remains below several major first-year alcohol findings.

Project MATCH approached eighty percent.

COMBINE reached nearly eighty-seven percent in some treatment groups.

And the instability does not wait five years to reveal itself.

It does not wait for chronic disease to reach its most expensive stage.

It does not wait for the next hospitalization.

The disability claim.

The lost job.

The depleted retirement account.

The next treatment admission.

Or the next generation to absorb the consequences.

A substantial portion of the instability becomes visible before the first anniversary of treatment.

Sometimes within months.

Sometimes within weeks.

Sometimes within days.

That is precisely the period in which the formal treatment episode has already ended.

The discharge has been completed.

The completion rate has already been counted.

The satisfaction survey has already been collected.

The outcome at the exit door has already been recorded.

The bed has already been filled again.

And the person has been moved into a category that sounds as though something has been successfully completed.

Alumni.

The significance of these findings is not that every person returns to use.

It is not that every treatment organization produces the same outcome.

And it is not that treatment produces no benefit.

Treatment can stabilize.

It can interrupt acute risk.

It can create a period in which recovery becomes possible.

The question is what happens after that stabilization is produced.

Because much of the evidence necessary to determine whether treatment became durable lies precisely in the period the treatment system routinely stops measuring.

The problem is therefore not simply that recurrence occurs after discharge.

It is that the system can define success before the period in which durability can actually be tested.

The person returning to opioid use within a week is someone's alumnus.

The person unable to sustain methamphetamine abstinence through the first year is someone's alumnus.

The person drinking again six months after treatment is someone's alumnus.

The person represented inside the seventy-percent economic model is someone's alumnus.

The person represented inside the seventy-five-percent Project MATCH finding is someone's alumnus.

The person represented inside the COMBINE treatment arms where more than eighty percent experienced heavy drinking again is someone's alumnus.

The statistics may appear in different studies.

The people do not disappear into them.

Every one of these clients is counted among someone's alumni, often with no traceable evidence that the skills, capacities, or competencies required for durable recovery were ever developed.

The Kantian Indictment

Under Kantian reasoning, a system that measures only the treatment episode cannot legitimately claim that it produces recovery beyond it.

When a treatment program reports a completion rate, it is making a claim about a variable it has measured.

When it claims to produce recovery, it is making a claim about a variable it has not measured and, in many cases, has made a structural decision not to measure.

That distinction matters because the boundary of measurement determines the boundary of what the system can legitimately claim to know.

This is not a limitation of what can be known.

It is a limit the system has chosen to place on what it will know.

A chosen limit is not incidental. It is a decisive act. And once that choice is embedded in the financial architecture, the consequences extend beyond measurement.

They begin to shape what the system is organized to produce: admissions, treatment episodes, and discharges.

When that structure is financially rewarded, the system becomes economically aligned with a model in which durable recovery is not required.

The organization can succeed financially whether durable recovery occurs or not.

That is the structural problem.

Recovery may occur. But the organization can still claim success without being designed to produce it.

A system that neither measures durable recovery nor organizes itself to produce long-term recovery cannot legitimately define itself as an addiction recovery system.

It is an admission-discharge system.

At its foundation, this is much more than an epistemological problem.

It is an economic one.

Tracking long-term recovery is not free.

Longitudinal measurement requires infrastructure.

Follow-up staff, post-discharge engagement, data collection, and continuity all cost money.

Fee-for-service reimbursement does not reliably pay for them.

So the program that tracks what happens after discharge assumes costs that the program that does not track outcomes can avoid.

Ignorance is cheaper.

Incentive Structure

Consider the incentive structure.

Under fee-for-service reimbursement, still the dominant payment model for most addiction treatment services, programs are paid for delivering services.

They are paid for admission assessments.

They are paid for therapy sessions.

They are paid for medication management.

They are paid for discharge planning.

They are paid, in short, for activity.

They are not paid for outcomes.

They are not paid for the stability of their clients six months after discharge.

They are not paid for the recovery capital their clients have accumulated a year after treatment.

They are not paid for the reduction in chronic disease progression in their client population.

They are not paid for the rate at which their clients remain stably employed two years after discharge.

This is not because long-term outcomes are beyond observation.

Research studies and a small number of value-based contracting experiments already follow them, but those efforts represent only a fraction of the industry's total reimbursement.

Universal longitudinal measurement would also reveal the performance differential between programs.

That differential would create competitive pressure toward the investments required to improve outcomes.

Programs that measure their six-month post-discharge recurrence rates and disclose them publicly invite comparison.

Programs that invest in one-year recovery support infrastructure incur costs that programs relying on episodic reimbursement do not.

In a market where programs compete primarily on admissions volume, marketing visibility, and amenities rather than on longitudinal outcomes, the programs that invest in continuity are at a cost disadvantage relative to programs that do not.

The current financial architecture therefore creates a competitive incentive structure in which outcome avoidance is financially rational.

This is profitable ignorance.

Not a lack of information, but a maintained state that is more financially comfortable than the alternative.

The alternative is knowledge.

Once long-term outcomes are visible, the question becomes unavoidable: what, exactly, is reimbursement for treatment episodes purchasing?

That question changes the terms of payment. If reimbursement is meant to purchase recovery rather than the delivery of an episode, financial performance can no longer be separated from what happens after the episode ends.

That requires a different financial model, one in which the revenue structure of addiction treatment is organized around outcomes rather than transactions.

The question is whether a different financial model can actually change program behavior or whether the incentive architecture is too entrenched for payment reform to matter.

The evidence says it can.

When treatment organizations enter value-based contracts that tie reimbursement to defined outcomes rather than delivered services, their behavior changes.

The investment calculus shifts.

Infrastructure that was previously irrational, including alumni tracking systems, post-discharge coaching, and longitudinal outcome measurement, becomes financially justified because it is now rewarded.

One data point illustrates the magnitude of what changes when incentives align.

In a value-based arrangement with Independence Blue Cross, reporting on 2019 plan data indicated that 5.6 percent of 71 members treated at Caron Treatment Centers were readmitted within 90 days.

In the same analysis, six other in-network providers reported 90-day readmission rates ranging from 11.6 to 25.7 percent.

This result reflects a specific payer-provider arrangement rather than a universal benchmark.

It demonstrates what becomes possible when financial accountability extends beyond discharge and into outcomes.

The clinical approach remained constant.

It was not the defining variable.

What changed was the financial architecture.

The program had a reason to invest in the infrastructure that reduces readmission.

It did.

Incentives changed. Behavior changed. Outcomes changed.

This is not a theoretical argument for a different financial model.

It is a demonstration of what occurs when accountability extends beyond discharge.

The question is not whether improved outcomes are possible.

It is whether the system is designed to produce them.

The Episodic Economy

The financial logic of episodic reimbursement is, from within its own framework, internally consistent.

Programs are paid per episode.

The episode has defined parameters: a beginning, an end, a set of billable services, a discharge standard.

Programs that complete the defined services within the authorized duration and produce a discharge that satisfies clinical and administrative criteria are financially successful.

Recurrence, within this framework, is not a system failure. It is the next episode.

When a client who completed a thirty-day residential program returns to use six months later and seeks treatment again, the program that provided the original episode generates a new admission.

The revenue cycle begins again.

The services are redelivered.

A new discharge occurs.

A new episode has been billed.

The program's financial performance is not impaired by the recurrence.

In some respects, it is supported by it.

A stable recurrence rate among former clients provides a predictable readmission pipeline that supplements the new admission flow.

This is not a description of malicious intent. It is a description of incentive alignment.

The insurance industry pays for episodes.

Treatment programs deliver episodes.

Recurrence generates new episodes.

Each participant in the system performs rationally within the incentives it faces.

The aggregate output is a system that maintains the instability population rather than depleting it.

Aristotle would recognize this structure.

A chrematistic system, organized around the value generated by each transaction, has no intrinsic mechanism for managing the long-term consequences of the transactions it produces.

It is oriented toward the next transaction rather than toward whether the treatment already delivered produced lasting improvement in the person's life.

The addiction treatment economy is, in Aristotelian terms, structurally incapable of governing the problem it exists to address.

Not because its participants are indifferent to outcomes, but because the financial architecture within which they operate does not organize their incentives around outcomes.

The shift to oikonomia, a system organized around sustained stability rather than transactional efficiency, requires not a change of heart among treatment providers but a change in the financial structure that governs their incentives.

The diagnosis is not that the system is broken.

It is that the system is working.

It is producing exactly what it is designed to produce: episodic stabilization followed by predictable recurrence.

That recurrence generates intensifying cost across institutions that never see the other's balance sheets.

The system is sustained by a financial architecture that rewards the treatment episode but does not remain responsible for what happens after it ends.

Value-Based Care

The emergence of value-based care contracting in addiction treatment is still nascent and represents only a small fraction of total reimbursement.

It is the first structural acknowledgment that the episodic model's incentive architecture cannot produce the outcomes the system claims.

Value-based care, in its simplest form, ties some portion of reimbursement to defined outcomes rather than to the delivery of services.

In addiction treatment, the outcome measures most commonly used in early value-based contracts are short-term: thirty-day readmission rates, ninety-day engagement rates, sixty-day abstinence rates.

These are improvements over pure fee-for-service activity metrics. But they remain, in important respects, extensions of episodic thinking rather than departures from it.

A ninety-day outcome window still preserves episodic logic.

It is longer.

But it is still bounded.

And it remains disconnected from the twelve-month stability threshold that defines durable recovery.

A program can optimize for ninety-day engagement.

It can produce strong short-term outcomes through intensive management.

But it can do so without building the infrastructure that sustains recovery across time — housing, employment, family integration, medication continuity, identity.

The result is improvement without durability.

The Mental Health Parity and Addiction Equity Act establishes important protections against more restrictive treatment of mental health and substance use disorder benefits than medical and surgical benefits.

But parity does not itself create an outcomes-based reimbursement model or require longitudinal measurement of post-discharge stability. It changes access protections, not the underlying architecture of recovery financing.

Value-based care goes further by beginning to alter the incentive structure. But altering incentives within an episodic architecture does not resolve the underlying design problem.

The core architectural problem is that the default financial model of addiction treatment rewards the transaction.

It is organized around the episode.

It is not organized around sustained recovery.

As long as that remains true, the system will continue to produce episodic outcomes while using the language of recovery.

Until revenue is tied to twelve-month Recovery Capital accumulation rather than thirty-day completion, the system will continue to reward the episode instead of the outcome.

A Long-Term Recovery System

Kant's analysis applies with full force.

A system cannot claim what it does not measure.

And a system built on thirty-day billing cycles has made a differen decision:

not to be accountable for twelve-month outcomes.

This is not a limitation.

It is a design.

The architecture is the problem.

And architecture does not change because the problem has been named.

It changes when the system is rebuilt around the outcome it claims to produce.

Durable recovery cannot be legitimately claimed as the product of a system designed to end before sustained recovery can even be known.

If recovery is the claim, durability must be the standard.

PART VI

THE DURABILITY STANDARD

Chapter 19:

Recovery Capital

The question is straightforward: what does durable recovery actually require, and how would we know if a system was built to produce it?

Answering it requires identifying the conditions that make long-term recovery more likely and understanding what changes when those conditions are sustained.

A durable recovery investment would not eliminate the economic and social costs of addiction entirely.

It would reduce them at a rate proportional to the improvement in long-term recovery outcomes.

Even a thirty percent improvement in durable recovery rates across the treatment-engaged population would produce economic returns that substantially exceed the investment required.

The arithmetic is not complicated.
Neither is the design choice required to execute it.

What has been lacking is not the evidence, not the economic logic, and not the technology to deliver continuity support at scale.

What has been lacking is a governing philosophy with the clarity and the authority to name the design failure and demand its correction.

That philosophy is Recovery Beyond Discharge™.

And the structural standard it proposes is the durability standard.

The economic consequences of instability extend across insurance markets, workforce participation, tax bases, and generational wealth.

Each reflects a different mechanism through which the failure of addiction treatment to produce durable recovery translates into economic cost.

Now the analysis turns inward.

Toward the individual, toward the biology of recovery, toward the specific conditions under which durable stabilization occurs and can be sustained.

Recovery is not determined by abstinence alone.

It is determined by the accumulation of internal and external resources that make stability possible across time.

That construct is Recovery Capital.

It is the framework through which durable recovery can be measured, understood, and evaluated.

This is the turn from diagnosis to measurement.

Recovery Capital is not a prescription.

It is the standard by which durability is demonstrated or exposed as absent.

Recovery Capital, as a clinical and economic construct, was developed by Robert Granfield and William Cloud in their 1999 research on natural recovery, the process by which large numbers of people resolve addiction problems without formal treatment.

William White's work significantly advanced and popularized the framework, and subsequent research by David Best further extended it, demonstrating that recovery is not only a function of individual resources but of social identity, community integration, and access to supportive networks that reinforce and sustain behavioral change across time.

The consistent finding across this body of research is that resolution is not primarily a function of willpower or moral character.

It is a function of access to the internal and external resources that make continued substance use less viable and sustained abstinence more sustainable.

Recovery Capital is the aggregate measure of those resources.

Housing

Stable, safe, substance-free housing is the foundational recovery capital variable. Without stable housing, the physiological regulation, the sleep architecture, the social stability, and the daily routine structure that recovery requires are impossible to maintain.

Housing instability is one of the strongest predictors of treatment failure. Housing is not an amenity that makes recovery more comfortable. It is a structural precondition for recovery to occur.

Employment

Meaningful work provides income, structure, identity, and social connection.

It is a critical recovery capital variable.

Employment provides the daily temporal structure that reduces the unorganized time in which relapse risk concentrates.

It provides economic resources that reduce the financial stress that is a major relapse trigger.

It provides a social identity that is incompatible with active addiction.

The role of the competent employee is difficult to sustain alongside the role of the active drinker.

Employment is not the opposite of addiction. But it is one of the conditions under which sustained recovery becomes more probable.

Health

Physical and mental health stability is a recovery capital variable that is frequently underestimated in treatment planning.

It includes medication continuity, regular medical care, and the management of co-occurring conditions.

Alcohol use disorder interacts with chronic physical health conditions in ways that complicate both.

Addressing only the addiction without stabilizing the co-occurring physical health conditions leaves the person managing a system in which every physical health crisis is a potential relapse trigger.

Health is the platform on which other recovery capital dimensions are built.

Relationships

Stable, supportive, substance-free relationships are among the most powerful predictors of sustained recovery.

People with stronger prosocial networks, more stable family relationships, and meaningful community connection have better long-term outcomes than those who lack these supports.

Recovery that occurs in social isolation is fragile. Recovery embedded in relationships that reinforce and sustain it is durable.

Community

Access to recovery-supportive communities provides the social infrastructure that sustains recovery when formal treatment ends.

Those communities include peer networks, mutual aid groups, recovery community organizations, and civic belonging.

Community capital is where identity reconstruction is reinforced, where the recovering person is seen as more than their disorder, and where belonging replaces isolation.

It is the domain most directly built by sustained engagement over time and most directly destroyed by premature discharge into social isolation.

Recovery Capital alone, however, is not sufficient.

The presence of resources does not guarantee their effective use.

What determines whether recovery capital translates into durable recovery is the individual's capacity to regulate internal states and to reorganize identity in ways that make sustained recovery viable.

Psychological Regulation

Managing stress, tolerating negative emotional states without seeking chemical relief, and regulating the nervous system's response to threat and frustration are psychological capacities.

They are not recovery capital in themselves, but they are the mechanisms through which recovery capital becomes usable and durable.

They are also the capacities most directly impaired by addiction and most directly requiring time and support to rebuild.

Psychological regulation does not emerge from insight alone.

It develops through practice, consistency, safety, and repeated exposure to the experiences of successfully managing challenges without substance use.

Identity

Identity is not a form of recovery capital.

It is the structure through which recovery capital is organized and sustained across time.

In addiction, that structure does not disappear; it is maladapted.

It is shaped by environments where stability required vigilance, performance, and self-suppression.

What presents in adulthood is not a lack of identity, but a system of protective identities built to survive instability.

For many people in recovery, identity reconstruction is not the work of building something new.

It is the work of returning to what was interrupted.

The self that learned early to hide, to manage, to perform stability in an unstable environment.

The hypervigilant child who constantly reads the room.
The ones who became afraid of people and authority.
The ones who learned to seek approval and lost themselves in the process.
The ones who felt responsible for everyone else.
The ones who could not express emotions safely and learned to suppress them.
The ones who confused love with rescue or pity.
The ones who feared abandonment and would do anything to avoid it.

The Adult Children of Alcoholics and Dysfunctional Families framework names the same pattern in lived terms: roles children adopt to survive unstable environments, which persist into adulthood as identity structures rather than temporary adaptations.

Internal Family Systems describes the same phenomenon at the level of internal organization: protective parts that take on roles.

They were carrying what had no language and no safe place to land: grief, fear, anger, shame.

What those parts were managing does not disappear simply with abstinence.

Sustained recovery allows the time and space for that integration work to occur.

Not through insight alone, but through time, repetition, safety, and the consistent experience of moving through the world without needing to perform or protect in the same way.

As that happens, the conditioned behaviors of a survival-based identity begin to loosen.

They are recognized, and no longer followed automatically.

And behavior begins to align.

Not with fear, but with integrity and values.

Identity formation in recovery is not the assignment of new roles.

It is the recognition that the person underneath the roles was always there.

That recognition takes time.

It requires the kind of sustained engagement with the world that a year of continuous recovery begins to make possible.

And it is this that becomes the foundation on which housing, employment, relationships, and regulation finally hold.

Recovery Capital Across Time

.The economic argument for extending recovery support to one year and beyond is precisely calibrated to the Recovery Capital accumulation timeline.

Recovery capital does not accumulate quickly.

Housing stabilization requires sustained sobriety and sustained income.

Both are fragile in the first months of recovery and strengthen across the first year.

Employment stabilization requires the kind of reliable performance that an employer will recognize and respond to with continued engagement.

That performance is inconsistent in the early recovery period and more reliable as the year progresses.

Psychological regulation requires the kind of neurological repair that research documents as occurring across a twelve-to-eighteen-month timeline.

Authentic identity formation requires the kind of repeated lived experience of sustained recovery that is simply not possible in thirty or sixty or even ninety days.

The alignment between the one-year threshold and the recovery capital accumulation timeline is not coincidental.

It is biological and social reality expressed in a number.

At one year of sustained recovery, neurological regulatory functions have meaningfully stabilized.

The highest-risk post-discharge period has passed.

The behavioral routines of recovery have been repeated long enough to begin consolidating as automatic responses rather than effortful choices.

The social and professional identity of recovery has begun to take root. The economic stability that supports continued recovery has a foundation.

The Five-Year Threshold

At five years of sustained recovery, the probability of maintaining recovery into the subsequent year approaches eighty-six percent.

Chronic disease trajectories that were being worsened by active substance use have begun to stabilize or reverse.

Workforce contributions are at their most reliable and productive.

Family stability has had time to rebuild.

Financial assets have had time to accumulate.

The five-year recovery dividend is not a metaphor.

It is a statistical reality with measurable economic components.

The person at five years of sustained recovery has a fundamentally different economic trajectory than the person at five years of treatment cycling.

And that difference is measurable across insurance claims, workforce productivity, disability probability, nursing home entry timing, and asset accumulation.

The one-year threshold is not a clinical preference.

It is the point at which the biological, psychological, and social conditions for durable recovery have had time to consolidate.

It is the point at which probability shifts meaningfully in the direction of stability.

The investment required to reach that threshold is bounded. The cost of not reaching it is not.

That asymmetry is the economic argument for the durability standard.

Recovery capital accumulates across time, and that accumulation creates a series of economic thresholds as stability becomes more durable.

The one-year stabilization threshold is the pivot point of the economic argument.

After approximately one year of sustained recovery, the probability of continued recovery crosses the fifty-percent threshold and rises with each additional year of sustained recovery.

It is the time investment at which the probability of continued stability increases significantly enough to change the expected value of the treatment investment.

The Economics of Time

Consider the economics.

A thirty-day residential treatment episode that produces thirty-day abstinence but is followed by recurrence approaching the seventy-percent modeling threshold within six months has a specific expected economic value.

Under that conservative modeling assumption, it produces, on average, the partial costs of the capital flow sequence in seventy percent of cases.

Those costs include the ER visits that result from recurrence, the chronic disease acceleration that continues during the recurrence period, the insurance claims, and the productivity losses.

A one-year recovery support program that carries an individual across the threshold where continued recovery becomes more probable than recurrence has a fundamentally different expected economic value.

Beyond that threshold, the probability of continued recovery rises with each additional year of sustained recovery, approaching eighty-six percent by the five-year durability threshold.

That changing probability alters the expected value of the recovery investment: the value of a career trajectory not disrupted by disability, of a chronic disease course not accelerated by continued alcohol use, of an insurance premium profile not elevated by sustained high utilization, and of an asset base that is preserved rather than liquidated.

The difference in expected value between these two architectures is not a matter of degree.

It is a matter of kind.

The episodic architecture produces an escalating cost curve.

The one-year investment architecture initiates an expanding stability curve.

This stability curve is the economic logic of long-term recovery infrastructure.

It is the argument that addresses the objection most commonly raised against extended recovery support: the cost.

The cost of extending support from thirty days to one year is real. It is approximately three to five times the cost of the thirty-day episode. That is a significant investment.

But the relevant comparison is not the cost of the extended program versus the cost of the thirty-day program.

The relevant comparison is the cost of the extended program versus the lifetime expected cost of the risk trajectory that remains when a thirty-day episode ends without sufficient continuity.

When that comparison is made honestly, it includes the chronic disease costs, the disability costs, the insurance costs, the federal program costs, and the generational wealth effects.

On that accounting, the extended program is not more expensive than the episodic model.

It is dramatically less expensive.

The economic case for durable recovery infrastructure is not a case for spending more on addiction treatment.

It is a case for spending differently.

The concept of the durability ladder describes the staged economic return that accumulates as recovery capital builds across time.

The Durability Ladder

Rung One: Thirty Days

Acute stabilization. Neurological acute withdrawal managed. Initial therapeutic engagement established. The platform for recovery is set, but fragile.

Economic return at this stage: primarily the cost of the ER visit or hospitalization avoided by treating the acute crisis in a structured setting rather than an emergency one.

Rung Two: Ninety Days

Early consolidation. Neurological regulation improving but not stable. Relapse risk very high. Behavioral habits of recovery beginning to form.

Economic return: reduced rehospitalization risk during the acute post-treatment period, beginning evidence of insurance cost reduction through reduced ER utilization.

Rung Three: Six Months

Significant neurological stabilization.

The transition zone that the neurological research identifies as the period when the brain moves from early recovery toward functional regulation.

Return-to-use risk still present but declining.

The six-month threshold is where meaningful economic differentiation between episodic and durable trajectories begins to appear.

Economic return: measurable reduction in healthcare utilization, beginning of workforce stability dividend.

Rung Four: One Year

The critical threshold.

Continued recovery has become more probable than recurrence.

Neurological regulatory functions meaningfully stabilized. Behavioral habits of recovery consolidated.

Recovery capital across multiple dimensions meaningfully accumulated.

Economic return:
A significant reduction in acute care utilization.
Early reversal of chronic disease trajectory.

Meaningful restoration of workforce productivity.
An improving insurance claims profile.

Meaningful stabilization in the family system, reducing the ongoing risk of adverse childhood experience accumulation in children.

Rung Five: Five Years. Durable Recovery.

The probability of maintaining recovery into the subsequent year approaches eighty-six percent.

Economic return:
Substantial reduction in chronic disease costs.
Substantial restoration of workforce productivity.

A significant reduction in disability risk.
Meaningful reduction in insurance costs.

And sustained family system stability that alters the developmental conditions of the next generation by interrupting the transmission of adverse childhood experiences and reshaping long-term health, behavioral, and economic trajectories across decades.

Accumulating Returns

Each rung of the ladder represents a different economic return.

The returns compound not just because the individual is accumulating recovery capital, but because the system costs that would have been generated by the alternative progression are not being generated.

Every month that does not produce a hospitalization is money and time saved.

Every year that does not produce a disability claim is revenue maintained.

Every decade that does not accelerate dementia onset is Medicaid expenditure deferred.

The durability ladder is the economic argument made concrete.

It is the reason that the investment in one year of recovery support produces a significant return that justifies its cost.

The Architecture of Durability

Recovery Capital explains why recovery begins.

Capacity determines whether it can be sustained under pressure.

Identity determines whether it holds across time.

Because identity is what organizes behavior when no one is watching.

Durability is what emerges when all three are aligned.

Recovery Capital → Capacity → Identity → Durability

This is the architecture through which recovery either stabilizes or collapses.

It is not theoretical.

It is observable across time, across populations, and across economic systems.

Every return to use, every readmission, every episode of treatment cycling reflects a breakdown somewhere along this progression.

Not a failure of will.

A failure of structure.

The question, then, is not whether this architecture exists.

The question is whether it is being measured.

Because without measurement, there is no accountability for whether recovery holds beyond discharge.

And without that accountability, systems continue to produce instability while reporting success.

The failure of addiction treatment is not only a failure to build durability.

It is a failure to even attempt to measure it.

Chapter 20:
The Institutional Continuity Assessment™

The cost of instability does not concentrate in the treatment episode.

It appears afterward in the household, the workplace, the insurance claim, the repeated admission, the public balance sheet, and the next generation.

That is not an oversight. It is an architecture that rewards episodes and does not reward sustained outcomes across time.

The treatment system measures the episode. The economic consequences accumulate beyond it.

That creates two obligations.

The first is continuity: support that operates across the period in which recovery is actually built rather than only the period in which treatment is delivered.

The second is accountability.

Someone has to be able to determine whether an organization has actually built that continuity.

Not in the aggregate. Not through a national estimate.

In a specific organization, on a specific date, from that organization's own records.

A treatment organization can adopt chronic-care language. It can operate an alumni program, publish outcome intentions, describe a continuum of care, and speak fluently about recovery beyond discharge.

And it can do all of that without ever being required to establish whether any of it functions.

That isn't dishonesty. It is the lack of a standard.

For as long as continuity cannot be evidenced, it can only be endorsed.

And an endorsement costs nothing.

The Institutional Continuity Assessment™ makes the presence or absence of continuity demonstrable.

Every measurement system is a statement of values.

What a system measures, it signals that it values. What it declines to measure, it signals it is willing to leave unaccounted for.

The field measures admissions, length of stay, completion, and readmission. Those things are real. Each describes activity inside the program.

None of them describes what happens after.

The technology to measure differently already exists. Validated recovery capital instruments exist. Alumni tracking has been built by programs willing to build it.

What does not exist is the requirement.

So the gap is not technical.

It is a governance gap, and governance gaps are closed by instruments.

What the Assessment Asks

The assessment asks one question.

Does this organization possess the infrastructure necessary to sustain recovery beyond discharge and can it evidence that infrastructure from its own records?

The second half of that question has rarely been required of this field.

Programs have been asked whether they believe in recovery. Whether they offer aftercare. Whether they care about their alumni.

They have not routinely been asked to establish, from their own documentation, whether those intentions amount to an operating structure across time.

The assessment also draws a deliberate boundary around what that question means.

It asks nothing about modality.

The field has genuine diversity of therapeutic approach, including twelve-step facilitation, cognitive behavioral therapy, dialectical behavior therapy, motivational interviewing, EMDR, Internal Family Systems, medication-assisted treatment, and trauma-informed care.

The research supports multiple approaches. The choice among them is a clinical decision, made inside the organization by people qualified to make it.

The assessment leaves that decision alone.

It examines something different: whether the organization has built the structure to remain accountable for continuity after the treatment episode ends.

A program can use evidence-based modalities and have no meaningful post-discharge infrastructure.

It can employ skilled, compassionate clinicians and be unable to demonstrate what happens to the people it discharges across time.

It can care deeply about long-term outcomes while operating inside financial structures that make investment beyond the episode difficult to sustain.

None of those conditions establishes a deficiency in clinical care.

They establish something different.

A structural condition.

That distinction matters because treatment and continuity are not interchangeable.

Treatment can stabilize.

Treatment can interrupt acute risk.

Treatment can create the conditions from which recovery begins.

But the existence of excellent treatment does not, by itself, establish that the structure required to carry recovery beyond it exists.

That is what the assessment measures.

Why Independent Assessment Matters

The next question is whether an organization needs an external instrument to establish something it may already understand about itself.

An organization may know its operations extraordinarily well.

It may track former clients carefully, maintain sophisticated data systems, and understand exactly where continuity succeeds and where it breaks.

If so, the evidence should show it.

But knowing the answer and independently establishing the answer are not the same thing.

There is also a problem of perspective.

Inside an organization, continuity rarely sits in one place. Clinical leadership sees one part. alumni coordinators see another. operations, admissions, finance, and executive leadership see others.

Each may understand its function perfectly.

What remains unanswered is whether those functions form continuity when examined together.

Ask whether an organization has continuity infrastructure and the answer may be yes: it conducts outreach, maintains alumni programming, measures outcomes, coordinates transitions, and remains available after discharge.

The assessment asks something different.

Do those activities operate together as a demonstrable system of continuity across time?

That question does not test whether individual activities exist.

It tests whether they function as a system.

And even when an organization has exceptional information and an accurate understanding of its own structure, it is still making a claim about itself.

Independent assessment converts that claim into a determination established against a common evidence standard.

That distinction matters to a board. It matters in investor diligence. It matters to a payer. And it matters to a chief executive who may need evidence strong enough to govern against internal assumptions.

The ICA™ is not necessary because organizations are incapable of understanding themselves.

It is necessary because institutional claims and independently established findings are not the same thing.

And an independent finding requires more than a general judgment about whether continuity appears to exist. It requires defined conditions against which that claim can be tested.

The Five Structural Indicators

Five indicators. None measures philosophy. Each measures whether infrastructure exists and whether the organization can evidence it.

Post-Discharge Contact Rate

Whether the organization maintains structured, system-initiated contact after discharge, and the rate at which that contact completes. A program that cannot maintain contact cannot demonstrate longitudinal outcomes. Most have no reliable answer. That answer is itself a finding.

Outcome Measurement Window

How far beyond discharge the organization formally measures and documents outcomes. If measurement stops at discharge, the organization cannot demonstrate sustained recovery. It can demonstrate completion. Programs can substantiate only what they can measure.

Alumni Infrastructure

Whether alumni engagement functions as a structured continuity system or as voluntary community activity. A contact list is not infrastructure. A social media group is not infrastructure.

Relapse Visibility

How return to use becomes visible other than through readmission. A program that learns of relapse only when a former client comes back is structurally designed to undercount it. Absence misclassified as success is not success. It is invisible failure.

Incentive Alignment

Whether leadership performance, staff evaluation, compensation, and governance reward longitudinal outcomes or episodic throughput. Most organizations tie incentives to admissions, occupancy, and length of stay. When incentives favor admissions, the system stays episodic.

This is the most revealing indicator in the assessment, and the one organizations are least prepared to be asked about.

Each of the five indicators is scored from 0 to 20 against a controlled tier structure, with an evidence-sufficiency rating recorded beside it.

The five indicator scores aggregate into the Continuity Capacity Score™ (CCS™), a bounded 0–100 measure of demonstrated structural capacity.

Sufficiency is not a footnote. It travels with the score, permanently, and it constrains what the score is permitted to claim.

A finding resting on testimony does not carry the weight of a finding resting on documentation. The instrument enforces that distinction rather than leaving it to the assessor's judgment.

The Score, the Classification, the Determination

The CCS™ is not a probability. Not a forecast. Not a grade.

It is a bounded 0–100 measure of demonstrated structural capacity on a specific date, built from five 0–20 indicator scores.

The score produces a maturity classification describing where the architecture presently sits:

Episodic System, **Transitional System**, **Emerging Continuity System**, or **Longitudinal Recovery Architecture**.

From the classification and the evidence follows one of three determinations.

Structurally Aligned

A verifiable continuity architecture exists beyond discharge. Structured post-discharge contact, longitudinal outcome measurement, integrated alumni infrastructure, relapse visibility, and institutional incentives aligned with recovery outcomes across time. The determination reflects demonstrated structural capacity. It is not a prediction about any individual.

Conditionally Aligned

Meaningful continuity elements exist. Structural gaps remain. Clients may have access to support after discharge, but continuity is inconsistent, dependent on voluntary engagement, or shaped by factors outside the organization's control.

Continuity Exposure

Clients are discharged into environments where continuity is voluntary, fragmented, difficult to verify, or absent.

This determination does not indicate a failure of treatment.

It reflects a structural reality present across most of the recovery landscape: long-term outcomes are being entrusted to systems that were never designed to sustain them.

The determination verifies that exposure.

It does not create it.

And no one arbitrarily selects it.

The assessor does not choose an outcome and assemble evidence toward it.

The score follows the evidence.

The classification follows the score.

The determination follows both.

There is no part of the instrument where a preferred result can be entered.

That same discipline extends to the economic analysis.

Continuity Economics

An economic argument requires an economic instrument.

This is where the two meet.

Using the organization's own records, the assessment produces a governed **Continuity Economics Exhibit**.

The Exhibit examines economic movement that ordinary institutional reporting can leave unresolved, including where demand comes from, what returns, and whether apparent stability reflects durable growth or repeated activity.

None of it appears on a financial statement.

Compounding cost. Repeat episodes counted as new demand. Referral relationships that appear durable and are not. Capacity that looks stable and is being refilled by the same people.

Ordinary financial reporting may accurately describe revenue, occupancy, acquisition activity, and enterprise performance while remaining unable to distinguish stability from recycled instability.

That is not an accounting failure. Financial statements were never built to answer the question.

The Exhibit asks a narrower one.

What can this organization actually substantiate from its own records?

An admission is a single recorded event. On its own, it does not establish whether the episode represents a first admission or a return to care, whether the person continued into further care, or whether the source that produced the admission reflects a durable referral relationship.

The Exhibit examines what ordinary admission reporting may leave unstated.

Where the evidence supports a conclusion, the finding is presented.

Where the evidence does not support one, the limitation becomes part of the record.

That second condition is the discipline that makes the first one credible. An organization that cannot produce its acquisition detail does not receive a blank space in the report. It receives a statement of exactly what was unavailable.

The gap becomes part of the record instead of disappearing from it.

The same discipline governs the limits of the Exhibit itself.

It does not value the business. It does not forecast performance. It does not produce a benchmark. It does not alter the score, the classification, or the determination.

It is corroborative, prepared under a controlled sequence that keeps it separate from the determination.

EBITDA can describe operating performance. Alongside ordinary financial and operating reports, an organization can see what it earned, what it spent, how full it was, and how efficiently activity converted into margin.

It cannot tell an organization whether the activity producing that performance reflects durable stability or recycled instability.

The Continuity Economics Exhibit examines that missing layer.

Not as a valuation. Not as a projection.

As a controlled examination of what the institution can substantiate from its own records.

How the Assessment is Conducted

The ICA™ is a remote executive structural review. On-site evaluation is not offered as part of the assessment.

Phase I: Controlled Evidence Review The organization submits documentation against a fixed evidence schedule. Every requested item reaches a recorded disposition, including the items that are never supplied. Evidence is reviewed for relevance, sufficiency, period consistency, and traceability. The assessor invents no evidence and supplies no evidence gaps.

Phase II: Leadership Architecture Interviews

Structured interviews across executive, clinical, and operational leadership examine how continuity is understood, implemented, measured, and governed. Testimony is evaluated alongside documentation. It does not replace it. Where what is said exceeds what is documented, the documentation governs.

Phase III: Structural Determination and Report

A controlled executive report presenting the Continuity Capacity Score™, evidence sufficiency, indicator findings, the Continuity Economics Exhibit, the maturity classification, and the structural determination.

The Instrument Measures. It Does Not Sell.

The assessment has to stop somewhere.

If the ICA™ identifies Continuity Exposure and then tells the organization what to buy, who to hire, or which provider to use, the independence of the determination collapses.

An evaluation that ended by naming what the organization should now purchase would be a sales instrument wearing the clothes of an assessment. Every board, every trustee, and every investor who has read a vendor-authored "assessment" knows precisely what weight to give one.

The ICA™ identifies and documents the structural conditions it finds. It does not select vendors, recommend specific providers, or make the determination contingent on any commercial solution.

What the organization chooses to do with that determination remains its own decision.

That separation is what gives the determination its credibility.

The ICA™ can establish what is missing without acquiring an interest in how the organization chooses to address it.

The Structural Answer

The determination identifies the gap.

It does not close it.

What closing it requires has already been established: continuity operating across the period in which recovery is actually built.

The problem was never that the field lacked language for this.

It had chronic-care language. It had recovery-oriented systems of care language. It had aftercare, alumni, continuing care, recovery management, and value-based care.

What it did not have was any way to determine whether those words described an operating structure.

That distinction is the whole of it.

Without an instrument, continuity remains aspirational. An organization can endorse it without building it.

It can describe activity without demonstrating architecture. It can point to outreach without establishing contact. It can point to alumni without establishing infrastructure. It can point to outcomes without showing how long they were measured, or who remained visible long enough to be counted.

And where the evidence does not exist, its absence can be explained away as an industry limitation rather than recorded as an institutional condition.

That is the escape route. It has been open for decades.

The assessment closes it.

It does not make continuity more important.

It makes the absence of continuity harder to conceal inside language and easier to establish from evidence.

A condition that remains abstract can be debated.
A condition established as an institutional finding has to be governed.

That is the threshold the assessment now creates.

What the Answer Actually Requires

The answer remains continuity across time.

Recovery Beyond Discharge™ is the governing philosophy that defines it.

A continuum is the operating structure capable of carrying it.

Not an aftercare program. Not a discharge plan. Not an alumni newsletter.

And here is where most of the field's response to this problem fails, including the responses offered in good faith.

The continuity field has answered the post-discharge gap with duration.

Twelve months. Great.

Twelve months of the same meetings, the same app, the same coaching cadence, the same check-in call every Thursday.

That is not architecture. That is a schedule.

Most programs treat month three the same as month eleven. Same content. Same delivery. Same accountability structure, as though the brain at day thirty were the same brain at month nine.

It is not.

Executive function, including impulse control, judgment, and decision-making, recovers gradually across months, not days.

The nervous system is still adapting to life without the substance. Stress reactivity and craving responses can remain elevated well beyond acute withdrawal. And the internal and external capacities required to sustain recovery, including emotional regulation, relationships, daily structure, environmental stability, and recovery capital, are still developing across time.

These are not recovery metaphors. They are biological timelines.

Which means the brain has categorically different needs at day sixty than at month eight.

Treating them identically is not merely inefficient.

It is structurally misguided.

Continuity is not created by extending the same intervention across a longer timeline.

The innovation is sequence.

Differentiated support, delivered in the order that recovery capacity makes possible.

Recovery does not deepen simply because time has passed.

Anyone familiar with twelve-step recovery understands the concept of being "dry," time passing without recovery evolving.

The same principle applies to recovery architecture. Some work requires capacities that earlier work is still helping to establish.

Stability, readiness, recovery capital, regulation, relationships, and identity develop at different rates. The architecture has to be capable of responding accordingly.

Sequence is not a design preference.

It is the prerequisite structure neuroscience suggests.

The First Structure Built to That Standard

Recovery Matters® was built around a different premise.

If recovery changes across time, the structure carrying it has to change too.

The result is not one program delivered for twelve months. It is a continuum whose architecture evolves with the person moving through it.

The work changes.

The depth changes.

The demands change.

The technology changes with them.

And progression is not simply a function of time served.

The architecture changes as the person changes.

That is the distinction.

The individual methods inside the continuum are not the invention. They draw from established bodies of evidence across recovery science, behavioral health, recovery capital, emotional regulation, relational health, and long-term behavior change.

What is new is their orchestration. Distinct forms of support are brought into relationship across time rather than delivered as isolated interventions.

They are not assembled as a collection of services. They are organized to work together, with the nature, depth, and delivery of support changing as recovery changes.

Not everything belongs at the beginning.

Not everything becomes possible at the same time.

And not every person becomes ready for what comes next on the same day.

The person does not have to keep pace with the architecture. The architecture keeps pace with the person.

The specific sequencing, progression logic, measurement architecture, intervention protocols, curriculum deployment, and technological orchestration that make that possible remain proprietary to Recovery Matters®.

But the governing principle is visible:

Recovery is not held by repeating the same support for longer. It is held by changing the support as the person becomes capable of something more.

Continuity Includes Medication

Recovery architecture is not only behavioral, relational, or environmental.

For some people, medication is part of the architecture that makes recovery possible.

Addiction medications and medications used to support mental health do not become irrelevant when a treatment episode ends. When medication remains appropriate, continuity requires more than having received it during treatment or leaving with a prescription at discharge.

It requires access that can continue. Coordination that can continue. A structure capable of recognizing that medication needs may change as recovery changes.

This is particularly important because medication continuity is often treated as a separate transaction from recovery itself. The treatment episode ends. The prescription is written. The person leaves. What happens next is left to another system, another provider, another pharmacy, or the person to navigate alone.

That is another form of episodic architecture.

Recovery Matters Rx™ was developed to address that point of discontinuity.

It extends the Recovery Matters architecture into medication access and continuity, including addiction medications and mental-health medications where appropriate. The purpose is not to make medication the recovery model. Medication is one component of a larger recovery architecture, and for some people it is a critical one.

The Continuum provides the longitudinal recovery structure. Recovery Matters Rx supports medication continuity within that structure.

Neither replaces the other.

The objective is not simply to ensure that medication was available during treatment.

It is to reduce the possibility that a necessary component of recovery disappears simply because the treatment episode did.

Medication continuity is one part of the larger obligation: the structures supporting recovery have to remain available across the period in which recovery is still being built.

That period matters.

Return-to-use risk is highest during the first six months after discharge, a period in which executive function may still be recovering, recovery capital may still be thin, and the structures required to sustain recovery outside treatment are still being established.

One year represents a different threshold.

After one year of sustained recovery, the probability of continued recovery crosses the fifty-percent threshold and rises with each additional year of sustained recovery.

By approximately five years of sustained recovery, the probability of maintaining recovery into the subsequent year approaches eighty-six percent.

Twelve months is not the product.

It is the territory the architecture was designed to cross.

And reaching the other side does not end the relationship.

Alumni continuity follows program completion automatically, and support can be renewed or expanded at any point afterward, not as a restart but as recalibration.

There is a completion.

There is no cliff.

Because the continuum is delivered remotely, it goes where the person goes.

Home changes. Work changes. Relationships change. Geography changes.

The recovery structure does not have to disappear because the setting does.

That matters because one of the most ordinary fractures in the existing system happens at precisely that boundary: **the person leaves an environment where recovery was supported in treatment or in the community and enters one where recovery has to be rebuilt, reestablished, or discovered for the first time.**

Recovery Matters® was built to cross that boundary.

It is not an adjunct attached to the end of treatment.

It is not twelve months of aftercare.

It is not an app stretched across a longer timeline.

It is a long-term recovery continuum where evidence-informed curricula, recovery capital, and advanced recovery technologies converge inside an architecture designed to change because recovery changes.

That architecture required a different starting point.

Beyond Reimbursement

There is a reason this did not emerge from inside the reimbursement system.

The problem is not simply what reimbursement will pay for.

The problem is what happens when the full model is not guaranteed from the beginning.

A recovery continuum is designed as a whole. It begins with a defined core, while additional supports may become appropriate as recovery progresses. **The capacity to provide those supports, however, must already exist.**

If what exists next depends on what will be authorized next, reimbursement is no longer merely financing recovery.

It is deciding which parts of the model are allowed to exist.

That is a structural conflict.

Episodes fit reimbursement because they are discrete, bounded, and countable. Long-term recovery asks for something fundamentally different: support secured across time and capable of adapting with the person moving through it.

Recovery has to determine what becomes available next. The payment structure cannot be allowed to dictate what survives.

That is why a model built around the actual arc of recovery could not depend on the financing system that produced the gap.

It had to be built outside of it.

Private pay makes that possible now because the full continuum can be secured before it begins.

But private pay cannot be where the idea ends.

If Recovery Beyond Discharge™ is inherently harm reduction, then continuity cannot remain available only to those who can purchase it privately. The larger promise is what becomes possible when recovery infrastructure reaches enough people, for long enough, to interrupt the recycling of instability at scale.

That requires a different financial proposition.

When this model moves beyond private pay, reimbursement will have to become investment.

Not payment for the next authorized service.

Investment in long-term recovery as a whole, committed from the beginning and judged by what that investment produces across time.

Because the economic opportunity is not simply to pay for more recovery support.

It is to invest in the conditions that make repeated instability less costly, less damaging, and less inevitable.

The infrastructure has to exist before its outcomes can prove its value. Financing has to make that infrastructure possible without dismantling the very thing it is meant to support.

Because twelve months financed one authorization at a time is not continuity.

It is the episodic system with a longer discharge date.

The New Standard

The diagnosis has been made. The economic structure has been traced. The durability standard has been defined. And the answer has been argued from the economics rather than asserted from conviction.

What remained was to make the distinction visible.

For decades, this field has been able to speak about continuity without having to demonstrate it.

It could describe aftercare, alumni engagement, continuing care, recovery management, and outcomes without an independent standard capable of determining whether those activities amounted to an operating architecture across time.

That is what the Institutional Continuity Assessment™ changes.

It does not create continuity.

It does not prescribe it.

It measures whether it is there.

And where it is not, the absence becomes an institutional finding rather than an aspiration obscured by language.

That distinction matters because the problem has never been simply that treatment ends.

It is what happens when the architecture ends while recovery continues.

People move forward without sufficient structure. Instability returns. Families absorb it. Employers absorb it. Payers absorb it. Public systems absorb it. Treatment receives another episode, and activity that appears new may carry the economic history of what was never sustained before it.

The cycle begins again.

That is the recycling of instability.

The ICA™ makes that architecture measurable.

Recovery Continuums are built to change it.

One is an instrument of accountability.

The other is an architecture of continuity.

They should never be confused.

An assessment cannot sustain a person through the months in which recovery capital is still being built.

It cannot change with a recovering brain, strengthen a relationship, stabilize an environment, or remain present when geography changes and the treatment episode has long since ended.

Only infrastructure can do that.

And infrastructure changes the economic proposition.

If instability compounds across time, sustained recovery can compound across time too.

Every recovery capacity that holds extends beyond the person who developed it.

Stability moves outward. Into households. Into employment. Into healthcare utilization. Into children. Into families. Into communities. Into systems that no longer have to repeatedly finance the consequences of the same unresolved instability.

It changes generations.

That is the other side of the economics.

For almost a century, we have known that recovery takes time.

What changes now is what follows from knowing it.

If the condition continues, the responsibility cannot end simply because the episode does.

The question is no longer whether we believe in long-term recovery.

It is whether we are willing to build for it.

Recovery is not an episode.

The infrastructure built to sustain it cannot be one either.

Continuity.

Measured.

Built.

Carried across time.

This is Recovery Beyond Discharge.

Chapter 21:
Addressing the Objections

Every structural argument generates structural objections. The economic case for durable recovery infrastructure has encountered a predictable set of counter-arguments across policy discussions, treatment industry conversations, and insurer negotiations. Each deserves a direct response.

Objection One: "We don't have the evidence for one-year interventions."

This objection conflates the absence of large-scale randomized trials evaluating a specific long-term recovery continuum with the absence of evidence for the conditions that sustain recovery. They are not the same thing.

The research evidence on recovery trajectories is substantial. Long-term recovery research, recovery capital research, and decades of follow-up data from addiction populations consistently demonstrate that recovery changes across time and that the probability of sustained recovery increases as stability is maintained.

What remains limited is research on integrated continuums designed specifically around that trajectory.

That distinction matters.

Twelve months is not the intervention. It is the period across which different evidence-informed supports can be sequenced as recovery develops.

Housing stability, employment support, medication continuity, peer support, family integration, and recovery capital do not become evidence-based only when delivered together under a single model.

The evidence exists across the components.

What has not yet been tested at scale is their orchestration as a deliberately sequenced recovery architecture across time.

The evidence gap is in the architecture, not in the conditions the architecture is designed to sustain.

Objection Two: "This is too expensive."

This objection rests on a comparison that excludes the most significant costs.

The cost of extending recovery support from thirty days to one year is real.

A comprehensive one-year recovery continuum costs more, per individual served, than a thirty-day residential episode. This is true

But the comparison is not between the cost of the short-term episode and the cost of the one-year continuum.

The comparison is between the cost of the one-year continuum and the cost of the risk trajectory that remains when a thirty-day episode ends without sufficient continuity.

When the chronic disease acceleration costs, the insurance premium increases, the disability claims, the long-term care expenditures, the Medicaid costs, and the generational wealth compression are included in the accounting, the episodic model is far more expensive than the continuity model.

The objection that durability is too expensive is only plausible when the costs of episodic failure are distributed across institutions that do not see each other's balance sheets.

When those costs are aggregated and the full capital flow sequence is visible in a single accounting, the investment case for durability is not close.

This is the economic argument.
The pattern is measurable.
The math is unavoidable.

Objection Three: "People have to want to get better. You can't force recovery."

This objection is true as a statement about individual psychology and false as an argument against structural investment.

No one has proposed forcing recovery.

The argument for extended recovery support infrastructure does not require overriding individual autonomy.

It requires making the conditions for durable recovery available to individuals who want it.

The question is not whether individuals have agency. They do.

The question is whether the system provides adequate conditions for that agency to produce the outcomes it seeks.

An individual who wants sustained recovery and has access to twelve months of structured support is more likely to achieve lasting recovery than an individual who wants the same thing and has access to thirty days of support followed by a list of meeting times.

A 2021 randomized controlled trial, the NavSTAR study, illustrated the effect of structured post-discharge continuity: three months of structured post-discharge patient navigation for hospitalized adults with substance use disorders cut 30-day readmission probability from 30 percent to 15.5 percent, and reduced inpatient admission rates across the full twelve months of follow-up.

The intervention did not override individual agency.

It provided the structured continuity that allowed agency to produce a different result.

Agency operates within structure.

The quality of the structure shapes the probability of the outcome the agency is seeking.

Arguing that structural investment is unnecessary because individuals have agency is equivalent to arguing that public infrastructure investment is unnecessary because individuals have legs.

Legs are real.

Roads still matter.

Agency is real.

Infrastructure still matters.

Objection Four: "The system is already overwhelmed. We can't expand what we're doing."

This objection frames the problem as a capacity problem when it is an efficiency problem.

The current system is not doing too little of the right thing.

It is doing a significant amount of the wrong thing, repeatedly cycling the same population through episodes that do not alter their outcomes, generating high acute care utilization, high readmission rates, and downstream costs distributed across the system.

A system redesigned around durability would not necessarily treat more people.

It would produce better outcomes for the people it treats.

The capacity required for a well-designed one-year recovery support program is not dramatically greater than that required for a ninety-day program at a top-tier treatment center.

The difference is in the deployment of that capacity: concentrated across ninety days in one model and distributed across a full year in the other.

Over time, a durability-designed system would reduce demand for acute care by reducing recurrence rates, freeing capacity for the individuals currently untreated.

The system is not overwhelmed by doing too much. It is overwhelmed by doing the same insufficient thing repeatedly.

Objection Five: "Insurance won't pay for it."

This objection is often true under the current reimbursement architecture.

And that is part of the problem.

An episodic payment system is naturally better at financing discrete services than at financing recovery infrastructure across time.

Parity law establishes important protections against more restrictive treatment of mental health and substance use disorder benefits than medical and surgical benefits. But parity alone does not create a reimbursement model for longitudinal recovery architecture.

Nor should the economic case for continuity depend on any single regulation, payer policy, or reimbursement reform surviving unchanged.

The larger movement toward accountability for outcomes remains important. But the structural question comes first:

What would have to be financed if durable recovery, rather than episodic activity, became the economic objective?

Objection Six: "Medication-assisted treatment is sufficient. We already have an evidence-based solution."

Medication-assisted treatment works.

It can reduce mortality, stabilize neurobiology, reduce overdose risk, support abstinence or reduced use, and make sustained recovery more possible.

That is precisely why it belongs inside recovery architecture.

But in an episodic system, medication can become the minimum replacement for continuity.

The treatment episode ends. Medication continues.

And because the most immediate biological risk has been reduced, the system can treat that as sufficient.

At least they won't die.

That becomes the threshold.

Survival matters. It is the prerequisite for everything that follows.

But survival is not the same thing as recovery.

A person can remain biologically stabilized while housing remains unstable, relationships remain chaotic, employment remains inconsistent, recovery capital remains thin, and the conditions that made sustained recovery difficult remain largely unchanged.

In that context, medication is doing exactly what it is capable of doing.

The limitation is not the medication. It is the architecture surrounding it.

For opioid use disorder, the distinction is especially visible because medication can so directly reduce mortality and overdose risk.

For alcohol use disorder, the most widespread form of addiction, medication can also support recovery for appropriate individuals.

But the same structural question remains: what carries the person beyond biological stabilization into the rebuilding of a life?

Medication can stabilize.

Medication can protect.

Medication can support recovery.

What it cannot do by itself is become recovery continuity.

When medication is treated as the endpoint rather than one component of a larger recovery architecture, the system has not created durability.

It has created maintenance.

That distinction matters.

Recovery Capital asks a larger question than whether collapse has been prevented.

It asks whether the person is developing the capacities, relationships, stability, identity, and resources required for recovery to hold across time.

Medication is not the alternative to that architecture.

For the people who need it, medication belongs inside it.

The Cost of Not Investing in Durable Recovery

The question, then, is not whether these objections are understandable.

They are.

The question is what the cost of accepting them has been and what it continues to be.

The counterfactual analysis asks a simple question: what would the economic picture look like if the treatment architecture had been designed around durable recovery rather than episodic intervention?

The question cannot be answered with precision. There are too many variables, too many individual trajectories, and too much uncertainty in the extrapolations required to produce a single definitive number.

But it can be answered in direction and order of magnitude, and both are significant.

Consider the population of individuals who cycle through multiple treatment episodes without achieving sustained recovery.

For each member of this population, the capital flow sequence unfolds to some degree: emergency department utilization, work interruption, insurance cost contribution, eventual disability or early retirement, late-life care costs, and asset liquidation.

The specific course varies by individual, but the statistical pattern is materially costly across each of these dimensions.

The lifetime cost differential between the episodic cycle and durable recovery is estimated at approximately $500,000 to $1.5 million per person.

The estimate aggregates repeated treatment episodes, disability-related fiscal impacts, alcohol-accelerated long-term care, and lost tax revenue across a lifetime horizon. The total varies with disease progression and life trajectory.

At scale, even a population measured in the low millions produces an aggregate cost differential in the range of one to three trillion dollars over a lifetime horizon.

By contrast, extending that same population into one-year recovery continuums at an estimated program cost of approximately $100,000 per person would require investment measured in the hundreds of billions rather than trillions.

The return on that investment is substantial.

The Surgeon General's report notes that each dollar spent on substance use disorder treatment saves approximately four dollars in healthcare costs and seven dollars in criminal justice costs.

Modeled benefit-cost analyses, including those summarized from Washington State Institute for Public Policy research, show that returns can vary widely by intervention and population. The results range from low single digits to substantially higher returns in certain modeled scenarios.

These are not forecasts of realized program performance.

They are the range within which the economics of stability already operate.

A defensible central estimate, using direct healthcare costs, disability savings, and reduced long-term care expenditure over a twenty-year horizon, produces a return of approximately seven to eight times the investment.

At an investment level measured in the hundreds of billions, the prevented costs extend into the trillion-dollar range.

That central estimate is conservative. It excludes generational wealth effects, reductions in adverse childhood experience exposure, and the restoration of tax revenue from a workforce that maintains productive capacity rather than cycling through disability.
Including those categories increases the return.

These figures are directional.

Their purpose is not precision.

Their purpose is to make the magnitude visible.

And the order of magnitude makes the point: the cost of not investing in durable recovery is not comparable to the cost of investing in it.

The failure to invest is not incidental.

It generates escalating costs that dwarf the investment required to prevent them.

The system that manages episodes while the health of the underlying population erodes is not managing the problem.

It is financing it.

Chapter 22:
Architecture Determines Inheritance

At its core, the argument is simple.

Architecture determines inheritance.

Not in the metaphorical sense. Not as a poetic observation about how the systems we build shape the futures we leave behind.

In the literal, economic sense: the design of addiction treatment infrastructure determines what the next generation inherits.

It determines what the daughter inherits from the father who either achieved durable recovery or cycled through episodes without it.

It determines what the tax base inherits from the workforce cohort that either maintained its productive capacity or eroded it through alcohol-accelerated chronic disease.

It determines what the federal balance sheet inherits from the demographic transition.

The Medicare trust fund depletes at a specific rate. Medicaid long-term care expenditure grows along a specific arc. Both are shaped by the chronic disease and disability outcomes generated by the treatment architecture of the preceding decade.

It determines what children inherit from the ACE exposure produced by the adult instability that their parents' treatment either resolved or perpetuated.

These inheritances are not abstract.

They are specific.

They are measurable.

They unfold along trajectories that are clinically familiar and economically predictable.

The A1C that climbs another point.
The liver enzyme that crosses the threshold that triggers the specialist referral.
The cardiovascular event that produces the hospitalization.
The disability that ends the career.
The long-term care that consumes the assets.
The inheritance that does not arrive.

This is not a sequence of unrelated events.
It is a progression structured by the architecture that preceded it.

These are the economic outputs of the architectural choices made in every treatment program's billing cycle, in every insurer's authorization review, in every policymaker's budget decision about whether continuity infrastructure is a priority or an aspiration.

Recovery Beyond Discharge™ is the governing philosophy that makes these choices visible, links architecture to economic outcomes, and refuses to accept predictable harm as the operating condition of a compassionate system.

The dual proof is complete.

Volume One established the ethical argument: when harm is foreseeable and systems disengage anyway, that disengagement is not harmless.

It is a design decision with ethical consequences.

Volume Two establishes the economic argument: when harm is foreseeable and systems disengage anyway, that disengagement produces costs that extend beyond the billing cycle and compound across time, systems, and generations.

It is therefore economically unsustainable.

Together, these two arguments produce a conclusion that is both ethical and economic:

A nation cannot finance chronic instability through episodic intervention.

When a system is both ethically indefensible and economically unsustainable, structural redesign is not a reform option.

It is the only available rational conclusion.

That redesign requires only that treatment leaders, policymakers, payers, researchers, families, and others with the authority to act recognize that the current architecture is a choice, not a natural condition, and that the consequences of that choice are visible, measurable, and no longer deniable.

We can choose to build differently.

And if better outcomes are the goal, no other choice exists.

EPILOGUE

Like a readmission, we have been here before.

Jake checks his blood sugar before his next drink.

182.

Maya calls. He'll let it go to voicemail.

No one records this moment.

No dataset captures it.

No outcome report includes it.

He doesn't know it, but his last treatment center was sold in a portfolio to a PE firm for $275 million.

Success.

The system did exactly what it was designed to do.

Stabilized. Discharged. Disengaged.

He is not an exception.

He is not yet among the 178,000 who didn't make it.

Like so many others, he remains.

Someone profited.

He and Maya continue to pay the cost.

REFERENCES BY CHAPTER

Chapter 1 — The Inversion of Prevention

Felitti, V.J., et al. *Relationship of Childhood Abuse and Household Dysfunction to Many of the Leading Causes of Death in Adults: The Adverse Childhood Experiences (ACE) Study.* American Journal of Preventive Medicine, 14(4), 1998.

Leung, J.Y.Y., Parker, K., Lin, E.Y., & Huckle, T. The Association of Parental or Caregiver Alcohol Use With Child Maltreatment: A Systematic Review and Meta-Analysis of Longitudinal Studies. *Addiction*, 120(9), 1724–1738, 2025. doi:10.1111/add.70055.

Bellis, M.A., Hughes, K., Ford, K., Ramos Rodriguez, G., Sethi, D., & Passmore, J. *Life Course Health Consequences and Associated Annual Costs of Adverse Childhood Experiences Across Europe and North America: A Systematic Review and Meta-Analysis.* The Lancet Public Health, 4(10), e517–e528.

Merrick, M.T., et al. *Vital Signs: Estimated Proportion of Adult Health Problems Attributable to Adverse Childhood Experiences.* MMWR, 68(44), 2019.

Fang, X., et al. The Economic Burden of Child Maltreatment in the United States and Implications for Prevention. *Child Abuse & Neglect*, 36(2), 2012.

Centers for Medicare & Medicaid Services. *National Health Expenditure Data*, 2023.

Chapter 2 — The Recurrence Economy

Centers for Medicare & Medicaid Services. *National Health Expenditure Accounts*, 2023.
Substance Abuse and Mental Health Services Administration. *Behavioral Health Barometer* and *Treatment Episode Data Set (TEDS)*, current editions.

Bellis, M.A., Hughes, K., Ford, K., Ramos Rodriguez, G., Sethi, D., & Passmore, J. *Life Course Health Consequences and Associated Annual Costs of Adverse Childhood Experiences Across Europe and North America: A Systematic Review and Meta-Analysis.* The Lancet Public Health, 4(10), e517–e528.

Merrick, M.T., et al. *Vital Signs: Estimated Proportion of Adult Health Problems Attributable to Adverse Childhood Experiences.* MMWR, 68(44), 2019.

Chapter 3 — The Demographic Structure

Alzheimer's Association. *2023 Alzheimer's Disease Facts and Figures.*
Genworth. *Cost of Care Survey*, 2024.

Centers for Disease Control and Prevention. Alcohol-Attributable Deaths by Age Group, National Center for Health Statistics.
White, A.M., et al. *Alcohol-Related Deaths During the COVID-19 Pandemic.* JAMA, 2022.

Chapter 4 — Normalized Risk

Substance Abuse and Mental Health Services Administration. *National Survey on Drug Use and Health*, 2022.

International Agency for Research on Cancer. *Alcohol Consumption and Ethyl Carbamate.* IARC Monographs, Vol. 96, 2010.

National Cancer Institute. *Cancer Stat Facts*, current edition.

Chapter 5 — The Illusion of Containment

Pfefferbaum, A., et al. Degradation of Association and Projection White Matter Systems in Alcoholism Detected with Quantitative Fiber Tracking. *Biological Psychiatry*, 65(8), 2009.

National Institute on Alcohol Abuse and Alcoholism. *Helping Patients Who Drink Too Much: A Clinician's Guide.*

Substance Abuse and Mental Health Services Administration. *Recovery and Recovery Support: Recovery-Oriented Systems of Care.*

National Institute on Drug Abuse. *Principles of Drug Addiction Treatment: A Research-Based Guide*, Third Edition, 2012.

Chapter 6 — The Compounding Argument

Centers for Disease Control and Prevention. *Excessive Drinking is Draining the U.S. Economy*, 2022.

McLellan, A.T., et al. *Drug Dependence, a Chronic Medical Illness: Implications for Treatment, Insurance, and Outcomes Evaluation.* JAMA, 284(13), 2000.

Chapter 7 — The Capital Flow Sequence

Arendt, Hannah. *The Origins of Totalitarianism.* Harcourt, 1951.

Arendt, Hannah. *Eichmann in Jerusalem: A Report on the Banality of Evil.* Viking Press, 1963.

Mental Health Parity and Addiction Equity Act of 2008, Public Law 110-343.

Chapter 8 — Alcohol and the Employed Adult

Substance Abuse and Mental Health Services Administration. *National Survey on Drug Use and Health*, 2022.

National Safety Council. *Substance Use Cost Calculator for Employers*, 2019.

Goplerud, E., Hodge, S., & Benham, T. (2017). A Substance Use Cost Calculator for US Employers With an Emphasis on Prescription Pain Medication Misuse. Journal of Occupational and Environmental Medicine, 59(11), 1063–1071.

Centers for Disease Control and Prevention. Alcohol-attributable mortality data by age cohort.

.

Chapter 9 — Insurance, Risk, and the Marketplace

Kaiser Family Foundation. *Employer Health Benefits Survey*, 2023.

Mental Health Parity and Addiction Equity Act of 2008, Public Law 110-343.

Final Rule: *Health Reimbursement Arrangements and Other Account-Based Group Health Plans.* Departments of Treasury, Labor, and Health and Human Services, 2019.

.

Chapter 10 — Fiscal Asymmetry

Social Security Administration. *Annual Statistical Report on the Social Security Disability Insurance Program*, current edition.

Medicare Trustees. *2023 Annual Report of the Boards of Trustees of the Federal Hospital Insurance and Federal Supplementary Medical Insurance Trust Funds.*

.

Chapter 11 — The Price of Time

Alzheimer's Association. *2023 Alzheimer's Disease Facts and Figures.*

Livingston, G., et al. *Dementia Prevention, Intervention, and Care.*

The Lancet, 2020.

Genworth. *Cost of Care Survey*, 2024.

Cerulli Wealth Management Research. *U.S. High-Net-Worth and Ultra-High-Net-Worth Markets*, 2023.

Chapters 12–14 — Three Generations / Same Family / The Classless System

No external citations required. Narrative chapters drawing on data established in preceding chapters.

King, M.L., Jr. "The Minister to the Valley." Southern Christian Leadership Conference, February 23, 1968.

Chapter 15 — The Chronic Epidemic

American Society of Addiction Medicine. *Definition of Addiction*, 2019.

National Institute on Drug Abuse. *Drugs, Brains, and Behavior: The Science of Addiction*, 2020.

World Health Organization. *International Classification of Diseases (ICD-11): Disorders Due to Substance Use*, 2022.

McLellan, A.T., et al. *Drug Dependence, a Chronic Medical Illness.* JAMA, 2000.

Chapter 16 — The Limit of the System

Centers for Disease Control and Prevention. Deaths from Excessive Alcohol Use, current data.
Centers for Disease Control and Prevention. *HIV Surveillance Report*, historical data.
Centers for Disease Control and Prevention. Drug Overdose Deaths, current data.
SUPPORT for Patients and Communities Act, Public Law 115-271, 2018.
Federal Trade Commission. *Self-Regulation in the Alcohol Industry*, 2014.

Substance Abuse and Mental Health Services Administration. *TEDS* and *N-SSATS*, current editions.

American Hospital Association. *AHA Hospital Statistics*, current edition.

Whaley, C.M., et al. *Private Equity Acquisitions of Substance Use Disorder Treatment Facilities and Patient Outcomes.* RAND Corporation, EP71197, 2024.

Fuse Brown, E.C., and Hall, M.A. Private Equity and the Corporatization of Health Care. *Stanford Law Review*, Vol. 76, 2024.

Chapter 17 — The Model

No external citations required.

Chapter 18 — Profitable Ignorance

Kant, Immanuel. *Critique of Pure Reason*, 1781.

Aristotle. *Nicomachean Ethics* and *Politics*.

Mental Health Parity and Addiction Equity Act of 2008, Public Law 110-343, and Final Rules, September 9, 2024..

Smyth, B.P., Barry, J., Keenan, E., and Ducray, K. Lapse and Relapse Following Inpatient Treatment of Opiate Dependence. Irish Medical Journal, 103(6), 176–179, 2010.

Chalana, H., Kundal, T., Gupta, V., and Malhari, A.S. Predictors of Relapse After Inpatient Opioid Detoxification During 1-Year Follow-Up. Journal of Addiction, 2016, Article 7620860. doi:10.1155/2016/7620860.

Brecht, M.L., and Herbeck, D. Time to Relapse Following Treatment for Methamphetamine Use: A Long-Term Perspective on Patterns and Predictors. Drug and Alcohol Dependence, 139, 18–25, 2014. doi:10.1016/j.drugalcdep.2014.02.702.

McKetin, R., Kothe, A., Baker, A.L., Lee, N.K., Ross, J., and Lubman, D.I. Predicting Abstinence From Methamphetamine Use After Residential Rehabilitation: Findings From the Methamphetamine Treatment Evaluation Study. Drug and Alcohol Review, 37(1), 70–78, 2018. doi:10.1111/dar.12528.

Project MATCH Research Group. Matching Alcoholism Treatments to Client Heterogeneity: Project MATCH Posttreatment Drinking Outcomes. Journal of Studies on Alcohol, 58(1), 7–29, 1997. doi:10.15288/jsa.1997.58.7.

Friend, K.B., and Pagano, M.E. Changes in Cigarette Consumption and Drinking Outcomes: Findings From Project MATCH. Journal of Substance Abuse Treatment, 29(3), 221–229, 2005. doi:10.1016/j.jsat.2005.07.001.

Maisto, S.A., Hallgren, K.A., Roos, C.R., and Witkiewitz, K. Course of Remission From and Relapse to Heavy Drinking Following Outpatient Treatment of Alcohol Use Disorder. Drug and Alcohol Dependence, 187, 319–326, 2018. doi:10.1016/j.drugalcdep.2018.03.011.

Anton, R.F., O'Malley, S.S., Ciraulo, D.A., et al., for the COMBINE Study Research Group. Combined Pharmacotherapies and Behavioral Interventions for Alcohol Dependence: The COMBINE Study: A Randomized Controlled Trial. JAMA. 2006;295(17):2003–2017. doi:10.1001/jama.295.17.2003.

Chapter 19 — Recovery Capital

Granfield, R., and Cloud, W. *Coming Clean: Overcoming Addiction Without Treatment.* NYU Press, 1999.

White, W.L. *Slaying the Dragon.* Chestnut Health Systems, 1998.

White, W.L. *Addiction Recovery: Its Definition and Conceptual Boundaries.* Journal of Substance Abuse Treatment, 2007.

Best, D., and Laudet, A. *The Potential of Recovery Capital.* RSA Briefing Paper, Recovery Science Research Collaborative, 2010.

Dennis, M.L., et al. *The Duration and Correlates of Addiction and Treatment Careers.* Journal of Substance Abuse Treatment, 2005.

Crews, F.T., and Nixon, K. *Mechanisms of Neurodegeneration and Regeneration in Alcoholism.* Alcohol and Alcoholism, 2009.

Adult Children of Alcoholics World Service Organization. *Adult Children of Alcoholics/Dysfunctional Families.* ACA WSO, 2006.

Schwartz, R.C. *Internal Family Systems Therapy.* Guilford Press, 1995.

Chapter 20 — The Institutional Continuity Assessment™

Dennis, M.L., Foss, M.A., and Scott, C.K. An Eight-Year Perspective on the Relationship Between the Duration of Abstinence and Other Aspects of Recovery. Evaluation Review. 2007;31(6):585–612. doi:10.1177/0193841X07307771.

See Chapter 19 for Recovery Capital sources.

Chapter 21 — Addressing the Objections

National Institute on Drug Abuse. Long-term recovery trajectory research.
White, W.L. Recovery Capital research.

Gryczynski, J., Nordeck, C.D., Welsh, C., et al. Preventing hospital readmission for patients with comorbid substance use disorder: a randomized trial. Annals of Internal Medicine. 2021;174:899–909. doi:10.7326/M20-5475.
Mental Health Parity and Addiction Equity Act of 2008, Public Law 110-343, and Final Rules, September 9, 2024.
Cerulli Wealth Management Research. *U.S. High-Net-Worth and Ultra-High-Net-Worth Markets*, 2023.

U.S. Department of Health and Human Services. *Facing Addiction in America: The Surgeon General's Report on Alcohol, Drugs, and Health.* 2016. And: Washington State Institute for Public Policy. Benefit-Cost Results, Substance Use Disorder Interventions, current edition.

Chapter 22 / Epilogue

No external citations required.

ACKNOWLEDGEMENTS

This work was built on the research, clinical insight, and advocacy of many people who came before it. The scholars and practitioners whose work appears in these references did not write for the purpose of being cited in an economic argument. They wrote because the problem demanded it. That consistency of purpose, sustained across decades, is what made this argument possible.

To William White, whose foundational work on recovery capital and long-term recovery trajectories gave the field its language.

To Vincent Felitti and Robert Anda, whose ACE study made visible what had been quietly absorbed by millions of families.

To A. Thomas McLellan, whose articulation of addiction as a chronic medical illness remains the clearest statement of the clinical problem this book addresses economically.

And to David Best, whose work on recovery capital, social identity, and community has been central to how recovery is understood in practice and without whom this work would not have taken its current form.

To the practitioners, counselors, coaches, peer support specialists, doctors, nurses, therapists, social workers, case managers, and all who carry this work, especially those who remain when the system disengages, this book is written in recognition of that gap and in the conviction that it can be closed.

My own family for everything carried, seen and unseen.

To all those whose lives this system has touched:
the Jakes, the Roberts, the Mayas,
and the families around them:

the mothers, fathers, brothers, sisters, and children whose lives are shaped alongside theirs.

Whose ordinary trajectories carry the full weight of an architecture that was never asked to account for what it produces.

You are the reason this argument had to be made.

About the Author

Orlando Andrews, MSLC, CARC, CPRS, is an author, recovery systems architect, and founder of Recovery Matters®, a company focused on the design and delivery of long-term recovery continuums and infrastructure.

He writes from inside the field and from lived experience. His recovery is not background to this work. It is the origin of it.

Orlando developed the Recovery Beyond Discharge™ Governing Philosophy after confronting a system he once believed in and outcomes he could no longer defend. That reckoning became the foundation of this series.

When Systems Let Go established the ethical case.

The Economics of Instability demonstrates that what is ethically indefensible is also financially unsustainable.

He lives and works in the belief that systems produce exactly what they are designed to produce, and that knowing better obligates us to build better.

Recovery Beyond Discharge™

A Systems Philosophy for Long-Term Recovery

Authored by Orlando Andrews, MSLC, CARC, CPRS
Formally articulated in 2026

Recovery Beyond Discharge™ is a governing philosophy for the design and evaluation of long-term recovery systems.

www.ingramcontent.com/pod-product-compliance
Lightning Source LLC
LaVergne TN
LVHW100726061126
851857LV00011B/416
9798995184744